METHYL MAGIC

METHYL MAGIC

Maximum Health through Methylation

Craig Cooney, Ph.D.
with Bill Lawren

Foreword by Kilmer S. McCully, M.D.

**Andrews McMeel
Publishing**

Kansas City

www.andrewsmcmeel.com

99 00 01 02 03 RDH 10 9 8 7 6 5 4 3 2 1

Library of Congress Cataloging-in-Publication Data
Cooney, Craig.
    Methyl magic : maximum health through methylation / Craig Cooney with Bill Lawren.
        p.   cm.
    Includes bibliographical references and index.
    ISBN 0-8362-3585-1 (hbk.)
    1. DNA—Methylation—Health aspects. 2. Nutrition. 3. Dietary supplements. I. Lawren, Bill. II. Title.
QP624.C66   1999
613.2'6—dc21   98-45810
                                                                    CIP

You should seek the guidance of a qualified health professional before implementing the diet and dietary supplement recommendations in this book. Anyone who has, or suspects they have, a serious illness should consult a physician before undertaking the *Methyl Magic* program. Vitamins, minerals, and foods can interact with prescribed medications. The *Methyl Magic* program in this book should not be used as a substitute for qualified medical care or used in place of known effective treatments for disease.

ATTENTION: SCHOOLS AND BUSINESSES

Andrews McMeel books are available at quantity discounts with bulk purchase for educational, business, or sales promotional use. For information, please write to: Special Sales Department, Andrews McMeel Publishing, 4520 Main Street, Kansas City, Missouri 64111.

To my parents,
to Blitzy,
to Paul,
to Kim,
and to choosing science and Nature over bureaucracy.

CONTENTS

Foreword   ix

Preface   xiii

Acknowledgments   xvii

CHAPTER 1
Methyl Magic   1

CHAPTER 2
Villains and Heroes   10

CHAPTER 3
The Methyl Power Test   18

CHAPTER 4
The Methyl Magic Program: Food   25

CHAPTER 5
The Methyl Magic Program:
Supplements   58

CHAPTER 6
The Methyl Magic Program: Exercise   73

CHAPTER 7
Alcohol, Smoking, and Methylation   76

CHAPTER 8
For Women Only   82

CHAPTER 9
  Life and Methyl Power   96

CHAPTER 10
  Heart Disease and Stroke   112

CHAPTER 11
  Cancer   124

CHAPTER 12
  Arthritis and Lupus   133

CHAPTER 13
  Other Diseases   139

CHAPTER 14
  Methyl Magic and the Mind   154

CHAPTER 15
  Aging and Longevity   167

APPENDIX I
  Methyl Power Shopping Trip   188

APPENDIX II
  Methyl Magic Recipes   209

APPENDIX III
  Methyl Resources   227

REFERENCES   229

INDEX   245

FOREWORD

by Kilmer S. McCully, M.D.

A book for the general reader, written in readable style by a prominent scientist working in the field of aging and degenerative disease, is a valuable asset for anyone concerned about disease prevention. In *Methyl Magic,* Craig Cooney has written an authoritative, interesting, and informative book about a complex area of biology and human nutrition that is increasingly recognized as vital to health and preventive medicine. The description of this fascinating area of biology and medicine is distilled into a prescription for maintenance of health and vitality during the older years of one's life. The advice in *Methyl Magic* is based on sound, well-documented information derived from extensive research in man and animals. Carefully interpreted and extrapolated from the published scientific literature, the discussions and descriptions of these research results are balanced and sensible.

The subject of this book is aging and degenerative disease. During the past decade a number of important, large-scale human epidemiological studies have provided powerful evidence supporting the homocysteine theory of arteriosclerosis, which is the most important degenerative disease in the population. Although evidence implicating elevated blood levels of homocysteine, an amino acid derived from protein metabolism, was first realized in 1968, it is only recently that human studies have produced a revolutionary new understanding of the origin of arteriosclerosis.

As clearly explained in *Methyl Magic,* homocysteine is an indicator of deficient methylation, and efforts to prevent arteriosclerosis are centered upon counteracting the harmful effects of this amino acid on arteries. Arteriosclerosis in susceptible populations originates from subtle, chronic deficiencies of the B vitamins folic acid and vitamin B_6. Together with vitamin B_{12}, these essential nutrients control the production of homocysteine from methionine. Populations that are deficient in folic acid and vitamin B_6 because of consumption of refined and processed foods depleted of these vitamins have increased levels of blood homocysteine and increased susceptibility to coronary heart disease, stroke, and arteriosclerosis.

The recommendations in *Methyl Magic* describe the dietary and supplemental strategies that are needed to keep blood homocysteine levels within the desirable range. One of the most important aspects of the dietary approach outlined in this book is the emphasis upon fresh, whole foods—fresh vegetables and fruits, whole grain cereals, fresh fish and meats—that supply the folic acid and vitamin B_6 needed to prevent elevation of blood homocysteine and susceptibility to arteriosclerosis. Elimination of refined and processed foods from the diet—white flour, sugar, white rice, excessive oils—is a key feature of an effective preventive diet. In this respect the *Methyl Magic* approach is eminently sensible and realistic, providing an interesting and tasty dietary alternative to the overly restrictive and unworkable diets advocated by adherents of the outmoded cholesterol/fat approach to prevention of arteriosclerosis.

In the discussion of the power of methylation to modulate and regulate homocysteine within the body, *Methyl Magic* takes the argument of the homocysteine theory of arteriosclerosis to the next logical step. If homocysteine levels increase and DNA methylation and other aspects of methylation decline with age, what can be done to prevent or delay this eventuality? The basic argument is that "Many people [particularly the elderly] will probably find that extra nutritional support [from supplements] is needed to keep homocysteine low." The four recommended supplemental programs include folic acid, vitamin B_{12}, vitamin B_6 in a multivitamin supplement, vitamin E, betaine, choline, inositol, and fish oil. Each of these nutrients has been proved to lower homocysteine levels and to prevent progression of arteriosclerosis, thereby preventing coronary heart disease. The inclusion of betaine and choline is in line with the guidelines established by nutritional experts in this field, as reviewed by the Food and Nutrition Board of the National Research Council in the new edition of *Recommended Dietary Allowances*. By regulating the supply of methyl groups to keep homocysteine converted to methionine and S-adenosylmethionine, this program promises benefits and protection beyond that achieved by an optimal diet alone. This is excellent dietary and nutritional supplement advice for older adults.

There are many indications that deficiency of methyl groups and deficient methylation of homocysteine are implicated in a wide range of disorders. The scope of these disorders extends from depression and mental illness to birth defects, allergies, and autoimmune diseases. In each of these cases, elevated homocysteine levels in body fluids indicate a deficient supply of methyl groups. While the rationale to boost these deficient methyl groups through diet and supplements addresses aspects of these many disorders, final proof of the effectiveness of this approach remains to be demonstrated in most cases. An exception is the case of neural tube birth defects, where increased folic acid intake through diet and supplements lowers risk dramatically by lowering homocysteine levels in mother and fetus. *Methyl*

Magic provides a useful review of the status of deficient methylation in the causes and origins of these wide-ranging diseases and conditions.

The discussion of deficiency of methylation in aging is particularly fascinating. While the basic process of aging is incompletely understood by medical scientists, deficient methylation of DNA and homocysteine have come to be recognized as basic elements in the cause of aging. The *Methyl Magic* approach agrees with the recent proposal that thioretinaco ozonide, a compound containing homocysteine, vitamin A, vitamin B_{12}, and ozone, is required for energy production by cells. The loss of thioretinaco ozonide from cell membranes has been suggested to cause accumulation of oxygen free radicals within aging cells and tissues, supporting the free radical theory of aging.

Methyl Magic is an important, useful, and informative book that focuses attention upon a basic nutritional and biochemical area of great importance to age-related illness. The advice concerning dietary improvement and nutritional supplementation is sound, reasonable, and promising for prevention of arteriosclerosis, mental disorders, disorders of immunity, and other degenerative diseases. Current and future scientific investigation promises to develop conclusive proof of the effectiveness of the methylation approach. In the meanwhile, readers of this book have the advantage of adopting changes in diet, nutritional supplements, and other beneficial measures that will improve their health and prevent age-related illnesses.

Providence, Rhode Island
October 1998

PREFACE

When I was a boy my family had a dog, a white German shepherd named Blitzy. She was a member of the family before I was born, and when I was a baby she even bit a neighbor or two in my "defense." One day I saw my father leaving the driveway with Blitzy in the back of the station wagon. When I asked my mother where they were going, she explained that Blitzy had a tumor and Dad was taking her to the vet to be put to sleep. Blitzy wouldn't be back, she said. I asked why the vet couldn't do anything about it, and Mom replied that nothing could be done. Even then, when I was only five years old, I had a hard time accepting that nothing could be done to keep our faithful Blitzy alive and healthy.

Blitzy's plight triggered the beginning of my interest in aging. As I grew a little older that interest deepened, for the most personal of reasons. My parents had always told me that high blood pressure runs in our family. In fact, my grandfather actually died of congestive heart failure brought on by high blood pressure. He was only fifty-three, but high blood pressure (the medical term in his case was "malignant hypertension") had swollen his heart so much that when he died it filled his entire chest! Both of my parents had high blood pressure (now controlled with medicine). This all meant that high blood pressure was inherited, and my sisters and I were next. By the time I was in college, my blood pressure was rising high enough—140/90—to ring the alarm bells of a twenty-one-year-old.

Blitzy's death and my family's chronic, deadly problem with high blood pressure ignited my childhood interest in aging. By the time I was twelve I told my dad that I wanted to be a biochemist or a biophysicist so I could figure out why we get old. I wanted to know how we could slow aging and prevent the terrifying and debilitating diseases that kill us.

I grew up viewing science as the key to understanding the aging process. I realized that all the discussion of time in relation to physics, metaphysics, and religion didn't seem to slow down aging by even a day. (Note that Einstein, despite his unique insight into the nature of time and space, still got old just like the rest of us.) And money, which can't buy love, can't slow aging either (not unless we put that money into research on longevity).

I concluded that in order to do something about aging (other than just "feeling good" about it), time and aging would have to be examined as technical issues in biology and biochemistry, not just as a philosophical issue. I earned a B.S. in chemistry at California State University at Hayward and a Ph.D. in biochemistry at the University of California at Davis. I came to realize how important it was to understand how our DNA and our genes controlled aging or allowed aging to take place. If we wanted to slow aging, I realized, we would need to protect DNA from harm. If we could understand the genetic determinants of life span, perhaps we could manipulate our genes and protect our DNA in a way that would provide the elusive key to extending longevity.

In graduate school my adviser, Professor Morton Bradbury, suggested that if I wished to focus on DNA and aging, I should study DNA methylation. I didn't know much about methylation at the time, and the common explanation in textbooks was that DNA methylation was a curiosity without a known function. But Bradbury and a few others thought that this simple act of biochemistry deep in our cells—the addition of what was called a "methyl group" to molecules of DNA—might be a key to the aging process. There were already telltale hints from animal research, where the Russians had shown that as animals age, DNA methylation declines. This was a tantalizing suggestion: that loss of DNA methylation and aging went hand in hand.

So in 1979 I began to study everything I could find on DNA methylation. It turned out there was a lot of information, but most of it was in short scientific papers. Even so, these papers made it clear to me that DNA methylation was indeed important in aging and probably equally so in age-related ailments like cancer and heart disease. If DNA methylation controls some basic aspects of genes, then losing that control in aging or aging diseases could be serious indeed. But the state of scientific knowledge was so fragmentary that it was like having a few pieces of a jigsaw puzzle without knowing what the overall picture looked like. Still, I could tell it was a big picture, and I knew I'd better clear a big space to lay out the puzzle.

Eventually it became apparent to me that diet was a vitally important factor in methylation, perhaps one of the keys to health, vitality, and longevity. Why? Because so many of the components of methyl metabolism were nutrients: folic acid, vitamin B_{12}, methionine, choline, betaine—all found in foods we eat, or should eat, every day. But I reasoned that if we were getting enough of these nutrients from a "normal" or "natural" diet, then we should be living longer, healthier lives. Obviously "normal," "natural" diets weren't doing the trick. So if we were going to slow aging through nutrition, we would have to increase the amounts of these crucial nutrients in our diets. Since it would be hard to do that just by eating more methyl-boosting food, I thought we would probably have to fortify our diets with the key nutritional supplements that would keep our methylation machinery working in high gear.

I began to formulate a list of supplements that would boost methylation. Gradually I came up with a combination of nutritional supplements and doses that I was willing to try on myself. Fortunately nothing on the list was dangerous for a normal healthy person. So I picked out an amount of each nutrient that should boost methylation beyond the level that we get from a typical diet. I went out to the health food store and bought the best brands I could find of the components on my list. I started taking these supplements in a regular, systematic way. Within a few months I could see that the experiment on myself was working. I was definitely on the right track. I lost weight and felt much more energetic, both physically and mentally. My blood pressure—the danger sign that had helped inspire me to take action in the first place—went down dramatically. Nagging aches and pains all but disappeared. I got fewer colds and minor illnesses. In short, I felt like a teenager again.

I'll describe these and other changes brought on by methylating supplements in much greater detail later on. For now let me just say that I went on to recommend my methyl-boosting formula to my family, friends, and co-workers. Most, if not all of them, experienced the same kinds of dramatic health and vitality rewards that I had. It seemed almost as if I had hit on a magic formula—*methyl magic,* to coin the phrase that has become the title of this book. Now it's time to share this formula with you. May it enhance your life as it has mine.

To your health!

ACKNOWLEDGMENTS

I wrote *Methyl Magic* so that as many readers as possible could share the better health and greater longevity that are the rewards of fine-tuned methylation. The book is the culmination of decades of work, during which many people shared their knowledge, their science, and their spirit with me.

My parents always encouraged me to pursue my education and my interest in science. Eventually they became some of the first volunteers for my methyl supplementation program—the same program outlined in this book. My wife, Kimberly Cooney, provided all-important support and encouragement.

Juliette Dunham, my high school chemistry teacher, helped me decide to be both a scientist and an artist. Morton Bradbury and Harry Matthews, my graduate advisers, introduced me to DNA methylation and gave me brilliant advice. But it was my good friend and colleague Paul Frankel—someone who appreciates the significance of methylation in maintaining robust good health—who first suggested that I write a book on the subject. Our many discussions and the passion he shares with me for this subject matter helped make *Methyl Magic* a reality.

I would also like to acknowledge several pioneers in methylation and genetics research whom I have had the privilege to know and in some cases to work with. These include Boris Vanyushin, Arthur Riggs, Robin Holliday, George

Wolff, Lionel Poirier, Laura Mays-Hoopes, and Kilmer Mc-Cully, all of whom have in one way or another helped to make this book possible. I also greatly appreciate the many people, both scientists and laypersons, who gave me feedback about methyl supplements and who encouraged me to make this information widely available.

While the manuscript was in progress I had the invaluable aid of comments from Kilmer McCully, Claire Cooney, Agnes Cooney, Louis Fink, Neil Cashman, Fred Madsen, Steven Clarke, June Quinn, and Nina Shandler. Others, including Saul Kent, Terri Mitchell, Catherine Bennett, David Harrison, and my many friends in the FDA, have done a yeoman's job in promoting methylation and longevity.

No book sees the light of day without the help of collaborators, editors, and agents. In many ways *Methyl Magic* started with a conversation I had several years ago with Bill Lawren, a terrific science writer who became my collaborator and helped me see the book through to the finish line. I owe much to my literary agent, Wendy Lipkind, and to Christine Schillig and Jean Zevnik at Andrews McMeel for believing in *Methyl Magic,* and for expending great effort to see the book through from manuscript to bookshelves.

CHAPTER 1

METHYL MAGIC

T o Melinda,* it seemed that some vital switch deep in her body had suddenly and mysteriously been turned off. At forty-five a woman who could once dance through the night without drawing a deep breath was now struggling to summon up the energy to make a business meeting or cook a meal. She was developing worrisome physical symptoms: chest pains, arthritis in her neck, and sudden, inexplicable numbness in her feet. Her memory was slipping so noticeably that she had to plant spare car keys all over her house. Perhaps worst of all was a nagging depression, the inescapable feeling that her body, her mind—indeed, her entire life—was slipping irretrievably into a long and terrifying downward slide.

Melinda went to doctor after doctor, therapist after therapist, guru after guru. She tried drugs, meditation, and exotic herbs. But nothing helped for long. Finally she found a young doctor who was on the cutting edge of a new and as yet unpublicized medical breakthrough. He gave her a simple blood test, and when the results came back, he said, "I think we've found the problem."

The test results indicated that her body had a low rate of *methylation,* a vital metabolic process that takes place in

---

* "Melinda" is a composite, hypothetical case designed from a variety of reports in the published literature, to illustrate that some conditions can be treated with nutrition, and in many cases the needed nutrients are methyl supplements.

every cell and in each of the body's vital organs. Without this crucial process, the doctor explained, life could not exist. If your hidden methylation chemistry is humming along at the right rate, he told Melinda, it should help preserve health and vitality. If it's not, it can mean disease, depression, even despair. If Melinda wanted to be well again, the doctor said, she would simply have to boost her methyl power.

But instead of a shot or a prescription, the doctor gave Melinda a short, precise list of natural methyl-boosting supplements. She easily found all these supplements on the shelves in a health food store and bought a month's supply for about $15. A month later it was as if Melinda had been given a new life. Her physical symptoms had disappeared, her black depression had lifted, and she had the energy of a twenty-year-old. She threw away her spare car keys and signed up for a tango class.

Melinda's life was restored and rejuvenated because her doctor had performed a feat of *Methyl Magic*. He knew that much like the twirling dance of DNA, methylation is a major and fundamental determinant of health and sickness, or life and death. Like a car out of gas, life without methyl power comes to a screeching halt.

In our bodies methylation takes place more than a billion times a second. Methylation happens when one molecule passes a chemical fragment to another molecule. These chemical fragments are known as *methyl groups*, which are carbon atoms linked to three hydrogen atoms. Passing methyl groups from molecule to molecule is the basic act of methylation, and the impact of methylation on the state of your health can be enormous. Think of methylation as a central control dial, like a thermostat or the master remote control that runs your other remotes. The setting of that dial can either make you sick in a dizzying variety of ways or help keep you in tip-top health and condition for the rest of your very long life.

The good news is that the methyl dial is readily accessible—you can set it yourself at a robust, health-sustaining position using only a few simple strategies. No starvation diets or tasteless food, no boot camp exercises, no unmanageable self-sacrifices, no new age mantras.

Although my own condition was not as drastically miserable as Melinda's, our stories are similar. In fact, my story, though less dramatic, may actually be just as powerful and even more useful. Why? Because (other than my moderately high blood pressure) I was not ill by any medical definition. So in taking advantage of *Methyl Magic,* I wasn't treating illness, I was actually striving for a state of maximum physical and mental health.

After seven years of taking methyl-boosting supplements, I'm like a new man. My body's been "reshaped": I lost twenty pounds (I'm five feet eleven and now weigh 145), and my old spreading belly magically migrated north to my chest. And all this with absolutely no change in my exercise habits. I still play golf and bicycle regularly—no more exercise than I did before starting methylating supplements, but with a great deal more stamina—but I don't pump iron or use exercise machines. At the same time, my painful case of "racquetball elbow" virtually disappeared, as did most of the miscellaneous aches that begin to plague us all in middle age. Perhaps most important, my problematic high blood pressure has gone from 140/90 to an average of about 108/72—well within the healthy normal range.

I've undergone some other positive physical changes as well, although they may not be as dramatic as those I've just mentioned. I get fewer colds—almost none, really. I used to have ugly dark circles under my eyes, the kind that say you're working too hard or spending too much time in nightclubs. These have disappeared. I had to use dandruff shampoo almost every day to control runaway dandruff. Now I have to use it only once a month. I used to get buildups of wax in my ears; now that wax has turned to oil, which is much easier to clean.

The physical rewards I got from boosting my methyl power have been paralleled by noticeable gains in mental muscle. I'm a scientist, so my brain is on call most of my waking hours, and it's vital to my work (to say nothing of my paycheck) that it's firing reliably on all cylinders. Since I began to take methylating supplements, I can work much longer without becoming mentally fatigued. Before I began my methylation program I would have periods hours long—sometimes an entire day—when I felt a little "fuzzy" or "spacey" and just couldn't think very well. Since I started taking methyl supplements this rarely happens, and when it does, it doesn't last long. I have much more mental stamina: I can get through even the most lengthy and intense meetings or conversations without fading or spacing out.

My ability to do mental tasks—which, after all, is how I make my living—has improved tremendously. Although I haven't noticed great improvement in memory, other people who've gone on the *Methyl Magic* program tell me that their memory is definitely better.

In short, during the seven years that I've been boosting my methyl power I've become a brand-new version of myself, perhaps the best possible version. And my intuition is that I'll preserve this new physical and mental vitality well into old age. In fact, it wouldn't surprise me a bit if I ended up beating Jean Calment's longevity record of 120-plus years—and that's without the cigars!

It's my bet that you'll be able to reap many of the same rewards I have and more. You may trim down and shape up. You may boost your memory and your mental alertness. You may shore up your immune system. You may help prevent heart disease, stroke, depression, obesity, osteoporosis, and arthritis. There is evidence to suggest that you may be able to help prevent some kinds of cancer. And you may find, with your doctor's help, that you can use *Methyl Magic* to help treat chronic fatigue syndrome as well as emotional disorders like depression, alcoholism, and some forms of dementia. Perhaps best of all, there's tantalizing evidence that suggests *Methyl Magic* can slow down the aging process and perhaps even increase your chances of living the maximum human life span of 120-plus years.

If science makes you shudder, if you're already convinced—or at least intrigued by the idea—that *Methyl Magic* can do for you what it's done for me, you may be eager to launch your own methyl-boosting program right away. If so, feel free to skip directly to chapters 4 and 5. There you'll find the *Methyl Magic* program laid out for you in a set of simple, easy-to-follow prescriptions for supplements and dietary strategies that will keep your methylation mechanics fine-tuned.

But if you'd like to know what *Methyl Magic* really means, and why your body should respond to a program that boosts your methyl power, then read the next few chapters first. There are more than fifty years of solid science behind my recommendations, and while I won't regale you with all of it, you will get a feel for what methylation really means and how it works deep in your body to provide the health benefits that hundreds of people have already enjoyed.

METHYLATION: THE MYSTERY EXPLAINED

Methylation: it sounds like something you once learned in a chemistry class and promptly forgot as soon as the class was over. But you would have done yourself a favor by remembering it, because the truth is that methylation is one of life's most basic and vital functions. It starts at the moment of conception (even before, actually) and continues, billions of times every second, until the day we die. It helps determine who we are, what we look like, how we behave. Equally important, methylation is a vital key to how we feel—physically, mentally, and emotionally.

Let's put it as simply as possible: *Methylation helps give life, and it can take it away. In fact, without methylation there would be no life at all.*

So what is methylation? Technically it starts with the small parts of molecules called methyl groups. A methyl group is a carbon atom with three hydrogen atoms attached to it. You might imagine a methyl group as a three-eared Mickey Mouse cap. Any other molecule that puts on this cap, whether it be a molecule of DNA or a protein molecule—any of the body's enormous inventory of molecules— is considered methylated. Methylation is a part of our body's machinery, so crucial a part that it has a name of its own: *methyl metabolism.*

Actually, methyl metabolism refers to the making of methyl groups and their passing from one molecule to another. You might want to think of this process as a group of children passing around and putting on that three-eared Mickey Mouse cap. Methylation happens in everything that's alive—sponges, birds, bees, chimps, mice, and humans. As we said, without methylation there is no life—*period.*

But just as your car can run low on gas (or that group of children with the three-eared Mickey Mouse caps can get tired of passing the caps around), your methyl metabolism can run low, too. Your body might manufacture fewer methyl groups, or the rate at which those groups are passed from one molecule to another can slow down. In some cases, normal, healthy methylation can make a wrong turn, so that methyl metabolism becomes diverted or inefficient. When any of those things happen, our health can suffer in an amazing variety of ways.

This is because methylation has such a tremendous number of jobs to do in our bodies. Methylation helps regulate the switching on and off of genes (technically this is known as *gene expression*)—one of the most crucial regulators of health and life itself. When gene expression goes awry the results can be horrifying: birth defects, cancer, and maybe even autoimmune diseases such as lupus. When other aspects of methyl metabolism go awry the downside can be equally terrible: heart disease, mental retardation, and diseases of the nervous system, among others. The relationship between methylation and some physical diseases can also be linked to such emotional problems as depression, probably because methylation helps the body produce and break down *neurotransmitters*. These are the chemical messengers that keep our brain cells talking to one another and to other vital cells in the body. For example, neurotransmitters are linked to cells in the immune system, which is one of our most powerful defenses against disease.

Methylation also helps mobilize fats and cholesterol so that our bodies can process them. Methylation moves fats around and eventually out of the body so they don't pile up in the liver, which may in turn help protect us against nasty killer diseases like liver cancer and cirrhosis. Perhaps equally important, methylation "flushes out" harmful fats and helps regulate our weight and keep fats from accumulating in our arteries.

But that's just the beginning of methylation's job description. Methylation is essential to the production of melatonin, which we need to regulate our biological clocks and keep our daily sleep cycle in tune. Methylation is the main way our body clears and eliminates histamine, which can cause inflammation, allergic reactions, and even asthma. Methylation also plays an important role in keeping estrogen levels under control. Many experts think that high estrogen levels in women can contribute to breast cancer.

Among the most important of methylation's many functions is the maintenance and protection of DNA, the basic stuff of heredity and of life itself. Adding methyl groups to DNA is enormously important in maintaining healthy cells. When DNA methylation goes awry, cells can become cancerous, age prematurely, or actually "turn traitor" and begin attacking other cells in our bodies. This "cellular treason" can lead to so-called autoimmune diseases like lupus or rheumatoid arthritis. In fact, as we'll see later on, it's methylation of DNA that guides life itself at the moment of conception. And while we're still nothing more than tiny embryos, DNA methylation is the primary process that gives each of our cells their job assignments, "stationing" them, as it were, in the liver, the lungs, and throughout the organs of our bodies.

That's still not all. Methylation of certain proteins is essential to their proper function. For example, *myelin basic protein,* a component of the "insulation" that surrounds our nerves, depends on methylation to help keep nerves sending the right messages throughout our bodies. Many other proteins need periodic repair, and methylation is essential for this crucial repair work. Some of these proteins are vital to the proper functioning of our brains and nervous systems—if they're not methylated properly, these proteins can fall into such a state of disrepair that they could eventually bring on several serious, even deadly, afflictions of the nervous system. These may include seizures, cataracts, and Alzheimer's disease.

Methylation, to put it in a nutshell, is vital to the healthy functioning of virtually all our bodies' cells. Why? Because it makes the *membranes* that surround each of our cells more fluid. This in turn allows better regulation of the flow of life-sustaining minerals like sodium and potassium into and out of our cells, so that a healthy balance of these minerals is maintained. In most people the fluidity of cell membranes decreases with age, and this loss of fluidity may be one of the features that defines aging itself. It's possible that maintaining membrane fluidity through adequate methylation might even slow down aging!

Obviously methylation is a key player in giving us life, keeping us healthy, and perhaps in enabling us to live longer, more vital lives. Scientists have known this for quite some time, but I still find it amazing that there's been so little discussion of methylation in the popular press and in the media. It's a shame, and we scientists bear much of the responsibility for not making the public aware of what we know. Part of the problem, as I mentioned earlier, is that methylation is such a ubiquitous process—it takes place, after all, in every single cell in our bodies—that scientists have for the most part studied it in bits and pieces. So the big picture has yet to see the light of day.

But the big picture—most of its features, at least—is known, and more and more pieces are being put in place every week. So now it's time to draw that big picture and to show how vital it is to maintaining your body and mind, even your spirit, in a state of great good health. Read on.

CHAPTER 2

VILLAINS AND HEROES

In many ways our bodies are battlegrounds, hotbeds of
agitation and little wars that go on constantly, whether
we're aware of them or not. There are "good guys" and
"bad guys" fighting these wars: "bad guy" cancer cells appear
and, for the most part, are "shot down" by "good guy" natural killer (NK) cells produced by our immune systems. In
other cases, as I've mentioned, normally "good" cells go bad
and start attacking other cells, sometimes bringing on autoimmune diseases like multiple sclerosis and lupus. Methylation and methyl metabolism also have their galleries of
heroes and villains.

HCY AND METHYLATION

Just as in the old western movies, it's fairly easy to
identify the "good guys" and "bad guys" in health and disease,
and particularly in methylation. In the western entitled *Metabolism at the Methyl Corral*, the ringleader of the "bad guys"
is a substance known as *homocysteine*. (This substance is often
abbreviated as HCY and will be used this way throughout the
rest of the book.) HCY is an amino acid. Many amino acids are
basic building blocks of protein, but HCY has a special task of
its own: it helps keep methyl metabolism running. Ironically,
until fairly recently no one paid HCY much attention; it was
thought to be a relatively unimportant by-product of the
breakdown of the proteins we eat every day.

10

But as early as 1962 the first telltale clues began to emerge to indicate that HCY was very important indeed. Those clues took the form of a disease called *homocystinuria*, a condition in which levels of HCY are dangerously high (more than 100 micromoles per liter of blood plasma). Discovered independently by scientists in Wisconsin, Pennsylvania, and Ireland, homocystinuria was shown to be associated with some cases of mental retardation, eye disorders, osteoporosis, and damage to blood vessels.

The latter was part of a dramatic medical detective story that actually began in 1933, when an eight-year-old boy was admitted to Massachusetts General Hospital. This poor kid was in very bad shape: mildly mentally retarded, he had recently developed severe headaches, was suffering from drowsiness, and vomiting frequently. The natural lenses in his eyes were dislocated, so that he was having trouble seeing well. Over the next few days his condition deteriorated dramatically—he got a fever, his blood pressure began to rise dangerously, he felt weak, and his reflexes were abnormal. Only three days after entering the hospital he died of a stroke, which was almost unheard of in a child so young.

After his death, an autopsy showed that the boy had severe *arteriosclerosis*—clogging and narrowing of the blood vessels. In this case the clogged blood vessel was the *carotid artery*, which supplies blood to the brain. That explained why he had suffered a killer stroke. But it didn't explain why a boy so young had developed arteriosclerosis, a disease usually associated with aging.

More than thirty years passed before the boy's mysterious death was explained. In 1965, a nine-year-old girl came to Massachusetts General—the same hospital that had seen the ill-fated boy three decades earlier—suffering some of the same symptoms. The girl's mother told pediatricians that one of the girl's uncles once had similar symptoms and that he had died in childhood. She also knew that the uncle's case was written up in the *New England Journal of Medicine*. Sure enough, they found the story of the boy who had died of a premature stroke in the journal's November 23, 1933, issue. As chance and fate would have it, it turned out that the young boy who had died thirty years earlier was indeed this little girl's uncle. The Mass General physicians gave the girl a simple urine test. The test revealed that she was suffering from homocystinuria, a disease defined by much higher than normal levels of HCY.

In 1968 these cases caught the attention of Dr. Kilmer S. McCully, now a pathologist at the Veterans Affairs Medical Center in Providence, Rhode Island. In reviewing these two cases, plus another childhood case with unusual metabolism, McCully came to the historic realization that there must be a connection between HCY and arteriosclerosis.

It turns out that homocystinuria—as well as a number of other diseases I'll list in a moment—are either a direct result of methyl metabolism gone awry or the result of too little methylation to compensate for defects in processing HCY. If the rate of methylation is too slow (not enough of those Mickey Mouse caps being passed around or being passed too slowly), levels of HCY in the body rise. Cells that are less able to methylate HCY (or convert it to the normal amino acid cysteine) simply "dump" the unmethylated HCY into the bloodstream. Once this happens, havoc can result, especially if HCY levels remain high. HCY is normally cleared by the liver, but the liver can handle only so much of this task.

HCY levels are usually measured in blood or in urine and expressed in units known as *micromolar*. HCY levels of 100 or more define homocystinuria. At the other end of the spectrum, 15 micromolar or lower is considered normal. Between 15 and 100 micromolar is considered "high"—high enough, in fact, to constitute a condition called *hyperhomocysteinemia*. While not as dramatic as homocystinuria, hyperhomocysteinemia can still be a risk factor for a number of diseases. This methylation disorder can be the result of genetic factors, poor nutrition, or a combination of the two. Just as homocystinuria definitely causes arteriosclerosis and numerous other diseases, hyperhomocysteinemia very likely leads to arteriosclerosis, heart disease, and a host of other ailments, including neurological and psychiatric problems such as depression, stroke, and peripheral vascular disease, rheumatoid arthritis, and others. In pregnancy hyperhomocysteinemia is strongly associated with early miscarriage and with birth defects even if the baby does survive and come to term. In pregnant women high HCY may play a part in bringing on anemia, preeclampsia, and other complications. In addition, rising levels of HCY are often an unwanted and dangerous feature of aging.

But HCY doesn't have to be let out of the individual cell to cause problems. HCY can be toxic inside the cells as well. High levels of HCY inside the cells may interfere with the normal function of vital proteins that keep cells healthy. Too much HCY can also inhibit methylation inside the cells. If methylation reactions are reduced a small degree, it may just make you sick or your cells "sick." But if these crucial methylation reactions are reduced too much, it can kill cells outright. In fact, animal experiments have shown that injections of HCY can cause localized cell death. On the other hand, many scientists now think that high accumulations of HCY can raise levels of a substance known as *S-adenosylhomocysteine* (*SAH*), which is involved in methyl metabolism, inside cells. Rising levels of SAH may lead to the opposite effect: instead of killing cells, it may help switch on genes, known as *oncogenes*, which can lead the cells to become cancerous.

Perhaps the best-known danger of high levels of HCY is the role it can play in the development of arteriosclerosis, or clogging of blood vessels, which can lead to heart disease and stroke. We've already seen what happened to the unfortunate boy who died of a stroke at the age of eight. Although no one at the time thought of examining his levels of HCY, there's little doubt—especially given the experience of his niece some thirty years later—that his HCY levels were dangerously over the top. Over the past thirty years, and especially during the past decade, scientists have found enough evidence to convince many of them that HCY is a more important risk factor for cardiovascular disease than cholesterol! This will be further discussed in chapter 10 on heart disease and stroke.

HCY, then, is an important indicator of our methyl status. It's like the red ink, the debt and deficit, on our methylation balance sheets. If HCY levels are too high, it means that something's amiss in our methylation machinery. Either that machinery is not working properly or it's struggling to compensate for other aspects of metabolism that are slacking off. When methylation is off, it can lead to a host of other problems, both physical and mental.

SAM AND METHYLATION

If HCY is the villain in the methylation process, the "good guy" is named SAM. SAM's actually just scientific shorthand for a substance called **S-a**denosyl**m**ethionine. Discovered in the early 1950s, SAM facilitates nearly all methylation reactions in our bodies. (You might think of SAM as the captain of that team of children passing around the three-eared Mickey Mouse caps.) SAM is the "active" form of methyl groups, a "high energy" form made from *adenosine triphosphate* (*ATP*), our cells' "energy currency," and *methionine*, another amino acid that we'll meet again later. SAM is found mainly inside our cells and our tissues, including the red cells in our blood. Small concentrations of SAM are also found outside cells, in the blood plasma, for example, and in the fluid, known as *cerebrospinal fluid,* found in our brains and spinal cords.

SAM's big job in the body is to give methyl groups to other molecules. SAM, in other words, is the philanthropist in the methylation process, the Daddy Warbucks of methylation. The molecules SAM methylates are vital, and the placing of methyl groups on those molecules has enormous consequences in preventing disease and maintaining robust good health.

Here's a short list of the beneficial effects that methylation via SAM produces in the body:

- SAM is essential for the manufacture of melatonin, the hormone that helps regulate the body's biological clock.

- SAM helps make adrenaline, one of the "fight or flight" hormones, which helps rouse us in time of danger and without which we could not have survived as a species.

- SAM is a major player in the synthesis of *acetylcholine,* one of the most important neurotransmitters.

- SAM is a crucial component in the body's manufacture of *carnitine,* which helps deliver fatty acids from foods to feed the "energy engines" (called *mitochondria*) inside our cells.

- SAM helps the body brew *creatine*, a key component in the energy reservoir system in our muscles. (In fact, creatine is considered so important in building muscle strength that many bodybuilders take it as a dietary supplement.)

- SAM is essential for the synthesis of lecithin, which helps "package" fats and move them to the muscles, where they're burned for fuel.

- SAM is in charge of clearing and eliminating histamine, one of the "bad guys" in inflammation, allergy, and asthma.

- SAM has an important part in the metabolism of *dopamine,* a neurotransmitter key in regulating our moods and overall mental state.

- SAM also plays an important part in the metabolism of estrogen.
- SAM methylates DNA. The methyl groups that SAM helps attach onto DNA are essential for maintaining our cells and organs in proper working order.
- SAM methylates the *G-proteins,* which carry messages inside our cells, especially cells in the retina of the eye.
- SAM also attaches methyl groups to myelin basic protein, which is essential to the healthy functioning of our nervous systems.
- SAM helps repair age-damaged proteins—including many in our brains. If this damage goes unrepaired, it may contribute to seizures, cataracts, and Alzheimer's disease.

That's a short list, but SAM also acts on a larger scale. First of all, it increases cell membrane fluidity, which as we noted earlier is important for our cells' proper functioning and for general health. SAM also helps mobilize fats and cholesterol so that they can be moved to where they're needed in the body or "dumped" (excreted) if they're not needed.

Deficiencies of SAM are linked with depression, neurological disorders, heart disease, and a host of other debilitating ailments. As we'll see later, SAM is an effective treatment for depression. But it's also a pain reliever (analgesic) and can help treat such troublesome diseases as osteoarthritis, cholestasis (a slowdown in the flow of liver bile) during pregnancy, and some kinds of liver disease. In fact, laboratory tests have shown that in some cases SAM can actually prevent liver cancer in animals.

So HCY and SAM play the respective roles of bad guy and good guy in the story of methylation. To put it another way, SAM and HCY represent our "methyl balance sheets." HCY represents "methyl debt," or "methyl red ink." If you're getting behind, the rise in HCY is like a "methyl deficit." The same thing is true if your body is suffering a shortfall of SAM. Either case—too much homocysteine or not enough SAM—can compromise health and set the stage for a wide variety of diseases.

The vital question, then, is this: How do we balance the "methyl ledger" so as to maintain our bodies in a state of maximum good health? The answer is surprisingly easy. We can help regulate the balance of HCY and SAM by using some simple strategies. What are these strategies? They all have to do with the foods we eat and the supplements we take.

CHAPTER 3

THE METHYL POWER TEST

By now you may be intrigued enough to want to know how your own methyl machinery is running. Luckily there's a readily available test that will give you a strong clue. It's a relatively sophisticated blood test, but the arrangements can be made in your doctor's office. In most cases, all you have to do is ask. But remember, *you do have to make a special request to your doctor, because this test is generally not part of a routine physical exam.*

The test, known as the *fasting plasma homocysteine test,* measures the "total" HCY in your blood plasma from blood collected in the morning, before you eat. Your doctor needs to draw only a few milliliters of blood into a tube about the size of your finger. The blood is immediately separated into plasma and cells. The plasma is drawn off and frozen, then shipped to a testing laboratory where HCY will be measured using a high-tech process called *high-pressure liquid chromatography (HPLC)* or by a much newer process that's less expensive.

These processes are generally very accurate, but are time-consuming and thus can be expensive. A typical plasma HCY test costs about $30 to $100. Some insurance and health plans will pay for the present test. Some insurance pays for HCY tests only for people who already have had a heart attack. These are no doubt the same companies that pay for automatic barn door closers once the horse is gone.

HCY is a normal and essential part of metabolism,

just as cholesterol is. So it's okay, and probably necessary, to have some HCY in the blood plasma—just as it's normal to have cholesterol in the blood plasma. But high plasma HCY levels can be a warning sign. The HCY test is an excellent indicator of our risk for vascular disease, which in turn can help predict our risk for heart disease, stroke, or life-threatening blood clots. Although young women tend to have low HCY and rare incidence of vascular disease, the HCY test is still important for women in their childbearing years. Why? Because if HCY levels turn out to be high, then the woman is at risk for early miscarriage and complications of pregnancy as well as for delivering babies with neural tube birth defects.

The normal range of total HCY in blood plasma is about 5 to 15 micromolar. Even if your level falls in the "normal" range, remember that it's "normal" for many people to have vascular disease, and it's "normal" for most people to die in their sixties and seventies.

As the figure on page 20 shows, total plasma HCY levels can vary greatly. So ideally we should try to keep our HCY levels not just normal, but optimal. We don't yet know what "optimum" HCY levels are, although more research with an eye toward maximizing health and longevity should answer this question. But I recommend that people aim to keep their HCY at the low end of the normal range—say, about 8 micromolar or lower. Certainly if your HCY is 12 or higher, you'll want to at least take a multiple vitamin to keep it under control. Better yet, use the *Methyl Magic* formulas designed in large part specifically to keep HCY levels low in most people.

But let's say the results of your fasting plasma HCY test show your HCY levels to be in the normal range, yet you still suffer from vascular disease. Or perhaps you've had an early miscarriage, or a troublesome pregnancy marked by preeclampsia or anemia, or even the tragedy of a baby born with neural tube defects. In that case you may want to take a test that's even more revealing than the fasting plasma HCY

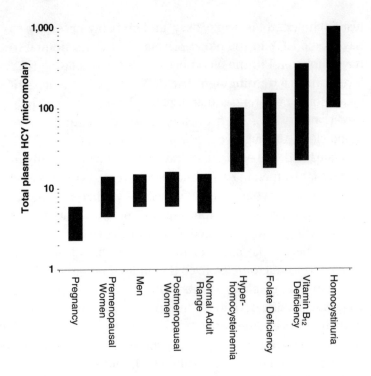

Total Plasma Homocysteine (HCY) under Various Circumstances
HCY levels vary greatly. HCY is lowest in pregnant and young women and highest in people with genetic or nutritional deficiencies such as homocystinuria and vitamin B_{12} deficiency. Note the steeply escalating logarithmic HCY scale. Adapted from Ueland, P.M., & Refsum, H. (1989), Plasma homocysteine, a risk factor for vascular disease: plasma levels in health, disease, and drug therapy. *Journal of Laboratory and Clinical Medicine* 114, 473–501.

test. That test is known as the *abbreviated methionine-loading test for plasma HCY.*

This is a more elaborate version of the HCY test. It measures how your methyl metabolism works under stress. For this test you have blood drawn in the morning before you eat, just as in the fasting HCY test. Then your doctor gives you methionine, usually in orange juice, at a dosage of 1 gram of methionine for every 10 kilograms of your body weight. Two hours later you get a second blood draw processed as in the fasting HCY test. The advanced test supplies you with more methionine than you would normally get in an entire day's meals. This in turn challenges your metabolism to recycle the extra load of HCY produced by the excess methionine. The methionine-loading test is more informative than the fasting HCY test. Unfortunately it's also more time-consuming and expensive—at least twice the cost of a normal HCY test. There's even a longer and, of course, more expensive version of this test, in which you receive several blood tests over twenty-four hours after a methionine load. But if you're generally healthy, your fasting HCY is low, and you already take methyl-boosting supplements, then these methionine-loading tests for plasma HCY may not be necessary.

Tests are also available to measure folates and vitamins B_{12} and B_6 in the blood. Again, if you're in good health, your fasting HCY is low, and you take supplements, then these tests may not be necessary. But if you suffer from depression, even mild depression, or have vascular disease, you may want to get tested for these methylating nutrients just to make sure the food and supplements you consume are enough to supply you with adequate blood levels of these substances. Also a combination of the HCY test and a blood test for methylmalonic acid (MMA) will tell you if folic acid and vitamin B_{12} are really doing their jobs in your body.

Remember that the lower end of the "normal" range for folates is almost certainly too low for keeping your HCY levels low and thus avoiding certain diseases, including depression. You'll probably want to keep your folate in the upper half of the normal range or higher. As a rule of thumb it's a good idea to keep red blood cell folate at 900 nanomoles per liter (400 nanograms per milliliter) or higher and keep serum or plasma folate at 12 nanomoles per liter (5 nanograms per milliliter) or higher. Your doctor can explain these values to you. Remember to take folate in combination with vitamins B_{12} and B_6 in the quantities recommended in this book: 800 micrograms folic acid, 500 micrograms of B_{12}, and 25 to 50 milligrams of B_6 (see chapters 4 and 5). The result will be lower, healthier levels of HCY.

LOOKING FORWARD

The present fasting HCY test measures "total" HCY in the blood plasma. But there's still a controversy among scientists as to what "total" really means. For example, many scientists are now looking hard at a form of HCY called *homocysteine thiolactone.* This is a natural variant of HCY and is a very reactive chemical that may modify our plasma proteins in a way that can't be measured by present HCY tests. This additional HCY may be important to measure in that it may be a greater or more specific risk factor for some diseases. Still, a large segment of scientists and the medical community would need to see research showing that this future test is a better indicator for risk of relevant diseases than is the regular HCY test. So it may be some time before the HCY thiolactone test shows up in your doctor's office.

The same may be true of two other revealing tests used at present in research laboratories. One of these measures blood levels of SAM. Because SAM is the means by which most methylation gets done, and is an indicator of several aspects of health and disease, it is important that it be measured in our blood. For patients with depression and other psychiatric disorders, blood SAM tests are especially important. SAM is often low in depressed patients, and elevating SAM can relieve depression. (For a more detailed explanation, see the section on depression in chapter 14.)

The second of these tests measures DNA methylation in the blood. For patients with autoimmune diseases like lupus, multiple sclerosis, or rheumatoid arthritis, white blood cell DNA methylation tests are important, because white blood cell DNA methylation is often low in individuals with autoimmune disease. Higher levels of white blood cell DNA methylation have been associated with improving autoimmune conditions. These tests are important because SAM gives us a good indication of the state of our methyl machinery, while white blood cell DNA methylation may give us a window into the levels of DNA methylation elsewhere in our bodies—which might be crucial in increasing our knowledge of and our ability to do something about cancer and aging.

Both these tests, SAM and DNA methylation, are used primarily in a research setting and are not yet widely available. Still, as time goes on and the importance of methylation becomes more apparent, these tests will undoubtedly help scientists understand and develop effective treatments for a wide range of methyl-deficiency diseases. The SAM test will be available soon. You can learn about newly available tests from the *Methyl Magic* Web site (www.methylmagic.com) and other sources listed in appendix III.

CONCLUSION

We know that moderate nutritional deficiencies, whether genetic or nutritional, can cause disorders in otherwise normal people. In fact, some people who test "normal" for nutrient levels and test "normal" in other ways still benefit from changes in their food and supplement intake. We don't yet know the optimal levels of plasma HCY, blood SAM, white blood cell DNA methylation, and so on. However, in the future the tests for HCY and blood SAM should become routine. You simply can't evaluate the real state of your health with great accuracy unless you can arrange to have these tests done. This doesn't mean, of course, that you can't be in good health without them. A personal program that calls for careful attention to what you eat, moderate exercise, and especially the use of *Methyl Magic* supplements will keep most people in good shape, at least by current, "normal" standards.

Let me repeat: The HCY test is currently available. If you want to get a glimpse of the real state of your health, it's important that you take this test. All adults, especially the elderly—remember that HCY levels tend to rise with age—should have their HCY checked. If it's high, then the *Methyl Magic* program is for you.

CHAPTER 4

THE METHYL MAGIC PROGRAM: FOOD

To get started on your *Methyl Magic* program, you need first to lay a good foundation. This means eating a healthy diet, one that will set the stage for boosting your methyl power.

So what constitutes a "healthy diet"? Obviously this is a loaded question with a wide range of possible answers, many of which are still controversial. Otherwise the bookstore shelves wouldn't be groaning under the weight of one diet tome after another—seemingly a new one every day.

As you probably know, many of these dietary prescriptions say flat out that people simply need to eat less food. Well, I have news for you: As the George Gershwin tune says, it ain't necessarily so. For many people, eating too much is less a problem than eating the wrong kinds of foods. This is especially true when you're trying to boost your methyl power. So the first and most basic trick in performing *Methyl Magic* is to take control of *what* you eat. Eat the *right* foods. In the process you'll eat *fewer calories* but probably a *greater volume* of food. In other words, eat the right foods and you can eat all you want—and still take advantage of *Methyl Magic*.

For example, a meal of pizza, soda pop, and ice cream probably doesn't have enough of the vital nutrients you need to keep your body working properly. But simply eating *less* pizza, soda pop, and ice cream (or just having a diet Coke with your pizza and ice cream) won't get you *more* of the vital nutrients you need—especially those that keep your methyl machinery humming along. So next time you go out for pizza, have a big salad and some lightly steamed mixed vegetables first. Then you'll probably eat less pizza, you'll almost certainly be full, and you'll at least have taken a step in the direction of setting yourself up to boost your methyl power.

Here are some tasty health guidelines on what to eat to lay that strong foundation for starting your *Methyl Magic* program. But remember, these guidelines aren't meant to be used just once or only for a month or two at a time. They're meant to be used every day (or at least 6.5 out of 7 days a week), as part of your normal routine. They're the rule rather than the exception. Taken as a whole, these *Methyl Magic* guidelines represent a change in culture—in your personal culture, my personal culture, and (hopefully) our culture on a wide scale.

FATS

In laying the dietary foundation for *Methyl Magic,* the most important consideration is fats—how much and what kind. Many people eat too much saturated and hydrogenated fat and too little of the essential oils that are the bedrock of a healthy dietary foundation. Because fats and oils are calorie rich (about 9 calories per gram, which is a lot—more than twice the calories per gram from proteins or carbohydrates), you want to be choosy. It's one thing if you blow the money for a haircut on your favorite horse or your favorite "get rich quick" scheme, but it's another if you do the same thing with the money for the mortgage or Junior's education. Likewise, don't blow your fat intake on a cow; invest it in an olive or a fish!

Most fats and oils contain a combination of saturated, monounsaturated, and polyunsaturated fatty acids. The important thing to pay attention to are the *proportions* of these fatty acids. In general, you want your diet to emphasize monounsaturated and some polyunsaturated fatty acids and deemphasize saturated fats, which come mostly from animal and dairy products and from tropical oils like coconut and palm oil, which are found in many prepared foods. Saturated fat raises blood cholesterol, and most people get too much in their diets.

On the other hand, vegetable oils (nonhydrogenated) generally, although not universally, contain more essential polyunsaturated fatty acids and smaller amounts of saturated fat than does animal fat. Some vegetable oils also contain generous amounts of monounsaturated fatty acids, and although these are not "essential," at least by today's definitions, they may have important and powerful health-promoting effects. In fact, these monounsaturated fats are thought to be one of the primary reasons there is significantly less vascular disease and cancer in Greece than in many other countries.

Many vegetable oils, nuts, and high-fat fish are good sources of monounsaturated and polyunsaturated fats. These fats are inherently more fluid, both in your kitchen and in your cell membranes, than are saturated fats. The fats in most fish are low in saturated fatty acids and contain rich quantities of omega-3 polyunsaturated fatty acids, which are known to have healthy effects on the heart and the blood vessels that feed the heart. (By the way, all oils I've ever seen contain some saturated fat. The labels on canola oil or products with canola oil that say no saturated fat aren't correct. But they still beat butter or shortening by a mile!)

A high-fat diet, especially a diet high in saturated fats, probably taxes methyl metabolism and probably raises levels of HCY, the "villain" (discussed in chapter 2) that can contribute to many diseases and poor health. On the other hand, oils found in many types of fish *lower* HCY and thus help pre-

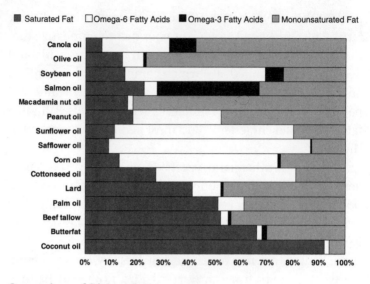

■ Saturated Fat　□Omega-6 Fatty Acids　■Omega-3 Fatty Acids　■Monounsaturated Fat

Comparison of Dietary Fats

Aim for a good representation of omega-3, omega-6, and monounsaturated fats in your diet. Using a combination of canola, olive, soybean, and fish oils achieves this goal. Some nuts are also high in monounsaturated oils (good) and low in saturated fat. Data and chart adapted from the USDA.

vent vascular disease. Epidemiological studies show that some cultures in which people consume significant amounts of fish—the Japanese, for example, or the Eskimos— have far less heart disease than those cultures consuming mainly cow fat (or other saturated fat). Also, our brains are largely made of the types of fatty acids found in fish oil.

Exceedingly important hormones in our bodies called *prostaglandins,* which among other things help regulate blood pressure, are also made from polyunsaturated fatty acids, including those found in fish. So if it's on a fish, it's fat you can have on your plate and eat without feeling guilty. I recommend eating fish at least two or three times a week. This way you may not have to take fish oil supplements as part of your *Methyl Magic* program. Of course, you could do both.

So here's a good rule of thumb for regulating the proportion of fats you eat to lay a good foundation for boosting your methyl power. Remember that the total fat in your diet should represent less than 30 percent of your total caloric intake. As much as you can, replace saturated fats with monounsaturated and polyunsaturated fat, so that your intake of saturated fat is less than 10 percent of your total caloric intake. You can achieve this by eating a diet that's very low in saturated fats. In other words, cut down your intake of meat, dairy products, and tropical oils, all of which are high in saturated fats. At the same time, increase your intake of monounsaturated and polyunsaturated fats by adding a *variety* of fresh canola, olive, soybean, and fish oils. Once or twice a week you may substitute nuts, avocados, or other sources of oil that are rich in monounsaturated or omega-3 polyunsaturated fatty acids.

But beware hydrogenated or partially hydrogenated vegetable oils, such as those in many margarines and shortenings. Unlike most other unsaturated fats, these oils contain a particular form of unsaturated fat known as *trans-fatty acids,* which have numerous health risks.

Note: In the following section, as well as elsewhere in the book, you'll see a few symbols. To avoid confusion, let's explain them here: CAF1 means carbohydrates as fiber. CAF2 means calories as fat. < means "less than." > means "more than." ~ means "approximately."

RECOMMENDED FAT SOURCES

Canola oil—contains essential fatty acids; use for cooking or fresh (for example, in salad dressings)

Olive oil—contains essential fatty acids; use for cooking or fresh

Soybean oil—contains essential fatty acids; use fresh

Fish—especially cold-water fish like salmon

ACCEPTABLE FAT SOURCES

Sesame oil

Most nuts (includes cashews, macadamias, peanuts, almonds)

Peanut butter

Sunflower

Safflower (high oleic preferable)

Avocados

Olives (black or green)

Generally NOT recommended foods: Consume rarely or only in small amounts. Small amounts of these after a full meal of the above healthier items can be okay. However, if you are trying to lose weight or just want to get control over your weight, you should avoid these. *Also, most of these provide a whole lot of fat and little of the folic acid and choline you need. Some of them are so loaded in fat that they aren't even a very good source of protein or methionine. In other words, these foods probably cause methyl debt and probably raise HCY!*

NOT RECOMMENDED FAT SOURCES

Hydrogenated or partially hydrogenated oils

Margarine

Shortening

Corn oil

Cottonseed oil

Palm oil

Coconut oil

Lard

Butter

Cream

Ice cream

Fatty meat

Chicken skin (unless fat is cooked out)

So that's the prescription for balancing your intake of fats to take maximum advantage of their power to regulate your methyl machinery. But fats are only one of the three major components (technically these components are known as *macronutrients*) of a healthy diet. The other two are proteins and carbohydrates. To lay the proper foundation for your *Methyl Magic* program, you'll want to pay as much attention to these dietary components as to fats.

PROTEIN

If you want to perform *Methyl Magic,* one of your most important props will be the protein in your diet. This is because protein contains the essential amino acid methionine, which is absolutely crucial in methyl metabolism, crucial for life itself. But too much methionine raises HCY in humans and has been shown in lab experiments to shorten the life span of rats. On the other hand, too little methionine will not only limit your methyl metabolism, it's also a known risk factor for colon cancer. The trick is to make sure you're getting the right amount of methionine. Although scientists haven't yet established optimal methionine requirements, those requirements are probably about 2 to 3 grams a day for the average person. You'll get that much methionine by eating a diet such as the one outlined in this chapter.

But methionine isn't the only essential amino acid found in protein. Other indispensable amino acids are lysine, threonine, tryptophan, leucine, isoleucine, valine, phenylalanine, arginine, and histidine. These and other amino acids from dietary protein are used in the body to make structural proteins, enzymes, some hormones, antibodies, neurotransmitters, and other important molecules, many of which have to be methylated in order to perform their functions properly.

Nearly all natural foods contain protein. Animal products like meat are good sources, but you must be careful about the amounts you eat, because they're often high in unhealthy saturated fats. Look at the meat you buy—the more white streaks, the more saturated fat. If you're a beef lover, buy select grade—it's lower in saturated fat than choice, prime, or other cuts.

Beans and peas provide a fairly good balance of amino acids, as well as lots of fiber and very little fat. Good examples include soybeans, kidney beans, navy beans, lima beans, peas, and lentils. Grains, fruits, and vegetables (leaves and stems) are generally not good sources of amino acid–balanced protein. Some food combinations such as beans with brown rice (or rice bran) are complementary and offer a better amino acid balance than either food alone.

Fish, chicken, low-fat dairy, and a few eggs are recommended protein sources that contain healthy quantities of methionine and are good sources of vitamin B_{12}—another crucial player, as we'll see, in performing *Methyl Magic*. So include appropriate amounts of these foods in your diet, then balance them with vegetables and beans.

RECOMMENDED PROTEIN SOURCES

Fish

Some kinds of fish, such as tuna fish, cod, swordfish, flounder, can have very little fat. Unlike much land animal fat, fish fat can be healthy, especially if it's from cold-water ocean fish like salmon or turbot.

Shrimp

Shrimp is an excellent source of nearly pure complete protein with almost no fat!

Soy-based Products

Soybeans and their products are often high in protein and high in fiber. Soy oil, like fish oil, contains essential fatty acids, so some of this is good, but remember to hold your fat consumption to less than 30 percent of the total calories in a meal.

These days soy can be made into a cornucopia of tasty foods. Just check out your health food store—or even the natural foods sections that are now features in most "mainstream" supermarkets. You'll find soy hot dogs, soy burgers, soy milk, miso soup, and more. If you have figured out how to make tofu taste good or how to enjoy it as is, that's great! Here are some soy products that have that elusive combination of health and good taste:

Yves Veggie Pepperoni Fat Free

Yves Veggie Wieners Fat Free

Yves Tofu Wieners Low Fat

Boca Burgers

Lightlife Gimme Lean!

Beans

Beans are high in fiber and have moderate amounts of protein. Most beans besides soy have little or no fat. Beans are an excellent way to increase the fiber and reduce the fat in your diet while still getting some protein.

Chicken and Turkey

Chicken and turkey should be eaten without skin.

Skim Milk and Other No-Fat Dairy Products

A huge variety of no- or very low-fat dairy products are available today.

ACCEPTABLE PROTEIN SOURCES

The following foods are okay, but don't base every meal around them (base most meals around the highly recommended foods):

Hot dogs with less than 30% of calories as fat, such as Healthy Choice Low Fat Franks: 22% calories as fat; Oscar Mayer Free Hot Dogs: 0% calories as fat

Lean red meats

Eggs

Frozen yogurt or other low- or no-fat ice-cream substitutes

Truly low-fat cheeses (less than 30% of calories as fat)

Truly low-fat yogurts and other dairy products (less than 30% of calories as fat)

Low-fat milk (20% of calories as fat)

NOT RECOMMENDED PROTEIN SOURCES

These are also saturated fat sources:

Fatty red meat

Conventional hot dogs (often these have 80% calories as fat!!)

Whole milk (47% calories as fat), "2%" milk (most brands 37% calories as fat!)

Cheese: Even low-fat cheese is suspect; read the nutrition facts label, not just the front label—conventional cheese can have 80% calories as fat (so if "low fat" on the label front means 50% calories as fat, leave it on the store shelf!)

Whole-milk yogurt or other high-fat dairy products

CARBOHYDRATES

Carbohydrates are generally considered the chief source of the body's energy. Some people still refer to carbohydrates as "starches," but the carbohydrate family also includes sugars, vegetables, fruits, and legumes.

There's quite a bit of controversy these days as to what proportion of carbohydrates in the diet is healthy. For years high-carbohydrate diets developed by Nathan Pritikin, Dean Ornish, and others have ruled the dietary marketplace. These diets tell you to get as much as 80 percent of your total calories from carbohydrates, especially so-called complex carbohydrates found in fruits, vegetables, and grains. Recently there's been a shift toward more moderate diets—the program outlined in *The Zone* by Barry Sears is one good example—in which carbohydrates (again, mostly in their complex forms) make up about 40 percent of total calories.

For methylation purposes, carbohydrates are most important because they supply two dietary essentials: in their complex form, carbohydrates are a vital component of the generally healthy diet we need to provide a springboard for *Methyl Magic*. In addition, many sources of carbohydrates—especially vegetables and legumes—supply the specific nutrients that help turbocharge your methyl power. This will be discussed in greater detail in a moment. For now, though, let's start with a list of preferred sources of carbohydrates that will help get your *Methyl Magic* program off the ground.

RECOMMENDED CARBOHYDRATE SOURCES

Vegetables

Most vegetables are high in fiber. Fiber is good for you in and of itself —it keeps your digestive tract clean, slows your absorption of fats, and helps satisfy your appetite so that you're less tempted to fill up on unhealthy foods. Most vegetables are high in potassium and *phytochemicals*—substances that help reduce DNA damage, among other things. Vegetables are also high in antioxidants and in methyl-boosting folic acid, choline, and numerous other vitamins. In fact, consumption of fruits and vegetables has been associated with lower levels of the "bad guy" amino acid HCY discussed earlier.

Most of the following vegetables are available year-round:

Alfalfa sprouts

Artichokes

Asparagus

Bamboo shoots

Beans

Beets

Bok choy

Broccoli

Brussels sprouts

Cabbage

Carrots

Cauliflower,

Celery

Chervil

Cilantro

Corn

Cucumbers

Dill

Eggplant

Escarole

Garlic

Ginger root

Jicama

Kale

Leeks

Lettuces

Mushrooms

Okra

Onions

Parsley

Peas

Peppers

Radicchio

Radishes

Seaweed

Snow peas

Spinach

Squash

String beans

Sugar peas

Sweet potatoes

Swiss chard

Turnips

Water chestnuts

Yams

Zucchini

Fruits

Most fruits have many of the same advantages as vegetables. Many people find fruits more pleasurable to eat, and they beat the heck out of soft drinks and candy. Consider the following:

Apples

Apricots

Bananas

Blackberries

Blueberries

Cantaloupe

Cherries

Dates

Figs

Grapes

Mangoes

Melons

Oranges

Peaches

Pears

Pineapple

Plums

Prunes

Strawberries

Watermelon

These can be fresh and/or dried fruits. They also tend to have antioxidants, folic acid, and other methylating ingredients. In general, fruits provide healthy quantities of fiber and next to no fat.

ACCEPTABLE CARBOHYDRATE SOURCES

Whole-wheat/whole-grain bread

Whole-wheat/whole-grain bagels

Whole-wheat/whole-grain crackers

Whole-wheat/whole-grain pasta

Popcorn

Whole corn

Oatmeal and other whole grains, such as barley, wheat, millet, and rice

Some cookies with fiber, including some made by Health Valley or Tree of Life

NOT RECOMMENDED CARBOHYDRATE SOURCES

These are carbohydrates without much fiber, vitamins, minerals, essential oils, or phytochemicals.

White bread

White biscuits

White bagels

Most cookies

Soda pop

White saltine crackers

Refined sugar

White flour

Potatoes

Potato chips

Sugared desserts

The bottom line? To lay that vital foundation for your *Methyl Magic* program, eat a wide variety of foods. Use mainly vegetables and some fruits as the "bedrock" of your meals. Eat large portions (four to eight servings per meal) of vegetables and fruits along with fish, beans, low-fat dairy, or lean poultry (one to three servings per meal). At least once a day, preferably some with each meal, get a serving of the recommended oils either by eating fish or by using canola, olive, or soybean oil in a salad dressing or dip. Sometimes nuts, sesame oil, peanut oil, or olives, for example, can be acceptable substitutes for these oils. Whole grains are fine but shouldn't be the "centerpiece" or the bulk of most meals.

Finally, avoid or at least minimize your consumption of the foods on the "Not Recommended" lists.

If you're interested in maximizing the methyl power of your diet, here are a few commonsense tips that will aid you:

1. Eat most of your vegetables first. If your parents didn't teach you this when you were a child, it's not too late to learn.

2. Be aware of where the fat is. If you put fat (butter, margarine, mayonnaise, and so on) on everything, then keeping track is a nightmare. If you're using fat in only a few of your food sources (salmon and salad dressing, for example), then keeping track is easy.

3. Chew your food well. You'll eat more slowly, digest your food better, and be forewarned when you're getting full.

4. Eat! Don't starve yourself. Just be choosy about *what* you eat.

These are the general rules for establishing a healthy diet that will be a platform for your *Methyl Magic* program. Now let's get a little more specific. This chapter contains two types of guidelines:

1. If you prefer to know which foods to emphasize, use the food type guidelines.

2. If you prefer to calculate how much of particular food types—carbohydrates, fats, and protein—to eat, use the food proportions guideline.

FOOD TYPE GUIDELINES

Each meal should have a substantial amount of complex carbohydrate, protein, and fiber. Often the complex carbohydrate and fiber can be in the same food. Beans are a good

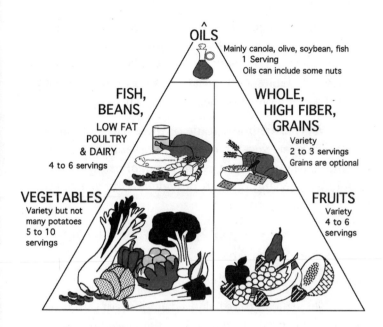

Methyl Magic Food Pyramid

The base of your diet should be vegetables and fruits. To make certain you get essential proteins and oils, you should add low-fat protein sources and specific oils—these appear higher up on the pyramid.

example of a single food that contains a good balance of nutrients. You should include small amounts (at least 2 teaspoons per day) of fresh canola oil, olive oil, or soybean oil. Balanced, complete meals are the key to building your *Methyl Magic* foundation.

Simple, good examples of such complete meals are the following:

Fish and vegetables: 4–6 ounces ocean fish; 10–14 ounces (or about 5 cups chopped) mixed vegetables (steamed or fresh), enough to fill ¾ of a standard 10-inch-diameter dinner plate; 3 ounces grapes (about 1 cup).

Chicken and salad: 4–6 ounces chicken (no skin); at least 10 ounces (at least 6 cups) mixed green salad, enough to fill at least ¾ of a standard 10-inch dinner plate; 1 tablespoon salad dressing (olive or canola oil–based); 4 ounces blueberries (about 1 cup).

You can combine some of these items in a mixture such as chicken vegetable soup; for example, Campbell's Chunky Hearty Chicken with Vegetable soup. Likewise, bean-based preparations can provide a well-balanced meal. For example:

Campbell's Healthy Request Split Pea with Ham soup

Health Valley Vegetarian Chili

Shelton's Turkey Chili with Beans

These meals have balanced amounts of carbohydrate, fiber, fat, and protein. Remember, the *proportions* are more important than the size of the portions. You can eat a lot—all you want, really—as long as you maintain the proportions indicated. You'll probably feel full and satisfied before you've taken in enough calories. If you still gain weight, increase the proportions of fiber and shift your fats more toward the healthy varieties.

FOOD PROPORTIONS GUIDELINE

Read the "Nutrition Facts" label on your food. This label is your friend, and can make figuring out a meal plan much easier. Once you do this a few times it should be easy. See diagrams on the following pages.

Carbohydrate as Fiber (CAF1): In your overall meal or snack more than 15 percent of carbohydrate grams should be fiber. On the "Nutrition Facts" label, find the grams of total carbohydrates and, under this, the grams of dietary fiber. Divide the number of grams of dietary fiber by the number of grams of total carbohydrates. (This is all the

Nutrition Facts

Serving Size 1 cup (240mL)
Servings about 2

Amount
Per Serving

Calories	170
Calories from fat	20
	% Daily Value**
Total Fat 2g	3%
Saturated Fat 0.5g	3%
Polyunsaturated Fat 0.5g	
Monounsaturated Fat 1g	
Cholesterol 15mg	5%
Sodium 480mg	20%
Potassium 500 mg	14%
Total Carbohydrate 28g	9%
Fiber 6g	24%
Sugars 6g	
Protein 9g	

*Percent Daily Values (DV) are based
on a 2,000 calorie diet.

Calculate CAF1

**(Carbohydrate as Fiber)
by dividing the Fiber Grams
by the Total Carbohydrate Grams,
as shown in the example below**

$$\frac{\text{Fiber Grams}}{\text{Total Carbohydrate Grams}} \times 100 =$$

$$\frac{6}{28} \times 100 = 21\% \text{ CAF1}$$

Note this food is high in fiber and passes the CAF1 test because it has more than 15 percent of carbohydrate grams as fiber.

Nutrition Facts and CAF1.

Locate the "Total Carbohydrate" grams and "Fiber" grams on the Nutrition Facts label and use them to calculate CAF1. If "Fiber" is separated into "Soluble Fiber" grams and "Insoluble Fiber" grams, just add these together to get your "Fiber" grams. In your meals you want CAF1 to average at least 15 percent.

---

fiber, both soluble and insoluble.) You can calculate this just as you would a 15 percent restaurant tip. Take the grams of carbohydrate per serving and figure 15 percent. You want the grams of fiber to be the same or greater than this. Twenty percent is even better. (Ask any waiter!) If the figure you come up with is less than about 0.15 (that is, 15 percent of carbohydrate as fiber, or CAF1), don't use much of the product. This is true whether you're going to eat it directly, as in a prepared or snack food, or whether it's part of a meal or recipe. Remember, a meal of beans and vegetables might have a CAF1 of 30 to 40 percent, while a fast-food meal of hamburger, fries, and soft drink will have a CAF1 of only 3 to 4 percent (or less).

Calculating the percentage of fiber is important only for foods that have significant amounts of carbohydrates. Let's say you're having a lunch of tuna fish, mayonnaise, whole-wheat bread, carrots, and an apple. After you gain a little experience you'll know that the carbohydrate and fiber sources are the bread, carrots, and apple. You don't have to bother calculating the CAF1 for the carrots and the apple because nearly all fruits and vegetables qualify. (The same is true, by the way, for meat, fish, or diet soda because they generally have little or no carbohydrate.) The important calculation is related to the bread. By choosing a bread that's high in fiber, and the proper amount, you keep the fiber/carbohydrate ratio high. This in turn gives you a tool to control your intake of calories. When your caloric intake is under control, you won't be wasting methyl groups on transporting excess fats around your body. Those methyl groups will then be free to help keep your HCY levels low.

Fiber isn't the only factor to consider when you're building a diet based on *Methyl Magic*. You'll want to be equally aware of your fat consumption.

Calories as Fat (CAF2): In your overall meal or snack, less than 30 percent of calories should be from fat or oil. On the "Nutrition Facts" label, find the calories per serving and then the calories from fat. Divide the number of calories from fat by the number of total calories. If this is greater than about 0.30 (that is, 30 percent of calories as fat), don't use much of the product. Again, this is true whether you're going to eat it directly, as a prepared or snack food, or whether it's part of a meal or recipe. (See Nutrition Facts and CAF2 figure.) A meal of beans and vegetables might have a CAF2 of 5 to 15 percent, while that fast-food meal of burger, fries, and soft drink weighs in at a CAF2 of 40 to 50 percent or more.

Nutrition Facts

Serving Size 1 cup (240mL)
Servings about 2

Amount
Per Serving

Calories	170
Calories from fat	20

% Daily Value**

Total Fat 2g	3%
Saturated Fat 0.5g	3%
Polyunsaturated Fat 0.5g	
Monounsaturated Fat 1g	
Cholesterol 15mg	5%
Sodium 480mg	20%
Potassium 500 mg	14%
Total Carbohydrate 28g	9%
Fiber 6g	24%
Sugars 6g	
Protein 9g	

*Percent Daily Values (DV) are based
on a 2,000 calorie diet.

Calculate CAF2

(Calories as Fat)
by dividing the calories from fat
by the total calories, as shown in
the example below

$$\frac{\text{Calories from fat}}{\text{Calories}} \times 100 =$$

$$\frac{20}{170} \times 100 = 12\% \text{ CAF2}$$

Note this food is low in fat and passes
the CAF2 test because it has less than
30 percent of calories as fat.

Nutrition Facts and CAF2

Locate the "Calories" and the "Calories from fat" on the Nutrition Facts label and use the formula to calculate CAF2. In your meals you want CAF2 to average less than 30 percent.

Let's use cooking oil as an example. If you're buying a bottle of canola oil, olive oil, or soybean oil, you'll be getting 120 calories from fat per 120 calories of product (in other words, 100 percent of calories as fat). If you're going to prepare meals with canola oil, you can control how much you put in your food. This can also be true of butter. You can sometimes use *very small* amounts of butter melted with canola oil or olive oil for added flavor. Use a small amount of butter in canola oil, for example: ¼ teaspoon of butter to ½ tablespoon of canola oil is a healthy proportion.

This calculation is most important for foods that contain a lot of fat. Let's go back to that lunch consisting of tuna fish, mayonnaise, whole-wheat bread, carrots, and an apple.

Once you get used to thinking of food in this way, you'll know that only the mayo might have too much fat. So control the amount of mayo you use so that your sandwich contains less than 30 percent of calories as fat. If you don't want to do the calculating, just follow this recipe, and you'll control the fat (there are additional recipes for a week's worth of *Methyl Magic* meals in appendix II):

TUNA SANDWICH

Ingredients
    Pickles (optional)
    Onion (optional)
    6 ounces tuna in water
    ½ tablespoon mayonnaise (soy or canola oil–based)
    4 slices whole-multigrain bread

Directions
    Finely dice pickle and/or onion; mix these with tuna and mayo to an even consistency.
    Spread on bread.

    Serve with apple, carrots, sugar peas, broccoli, and/or cauliflower.
    Makes 6 to 8 servings, enough for two sandwiches.
    This provides a fairly good balance of protein, carbohydrate, fiber, and fat.

    General rules:

1. You can use edible oils that are liquid at room temperature (especially canola oil, olive oil, fish oil, and moderate amounts of soybean oil).

2. If an oil or fat is *solid at room temperature,* don't eat very much of it (preferably none). Don't use hydrogenated or partially hydrogenated oils, coconut oil, palm oil, or cottonseed oil.

In your overall meal or snack, 20 to 30 percent of calories should come from protein. Vary your protein sources. Again, use the "Nutrition Facts" label. Be aware that meats and some fish are sources of a lot of fat. Be careful to choose very low-fat meat. If you eat a high-fat fish like salmon, you probably don't need other oil in that meal. Be aware that dairy products can be loaded with fat. You don't have to eliminate dairy products as long as the CAF2 in any given meal or snack isn't more than 30 percent. And you'll still want to get at least two-thirds of your fat calories from monunsaturated and polyunsaturated sources like olive oil, fish, or soybean and canola oils. All in all, your best bets for low-fat protein sources are fish, some other seafood (like shrimp), or beans.

By the way, you don't need to memorize all of this. Just take this book with you to the grocery store!

Note that in a low-fat food or meal the proportion of protein will be similar whether you calculate it using calories or grams. From the previous examples in the food types guidelines, here are calculations of percent protein, CAF1, and CAF2:

Split pea soup
Campbell's Healthy Request Split Pea with Ham Soup: ~23% protein (by grams), ~14% CAF1 (carbohydrates as fiber), ~12% CAF2 (calories as fat)

Chicken vegetable soup
Campbell's Chunky Hearty Chicken with Vegetables soup: ~30% protein (by grams), ~17% CAF1, ~22% CAF2

Chili
Health Valley Vegetarian Chili: ~32% protein (by grams or calories), ~47% CAF1, *no* fat

Most bean (no-meat chili) should meet the criteria (check the label to be sure).

Shelton's Turkey Chili with Beans: ~39% protein by grams (30% calories from protein), ~15% CAF1, ~15% CAF2

METHYL FUEL FOODS

Now that you've laid down the generally healthy foundation for your *Methyl Magic* program, it's time to focus on specific foods that contain fuel for methyl foundation. The following is a list of fuels, the vital ingredients in foods that help run your methyl machinery.

Choline: Choline is a methyl-intensive molecule. Choline has three methyl groups per molecule, or, if you like metaphors, three Mickey Mouse caps on. Choline is used directly by your body and needs no additional methylation. Your body also converts choline to betaine, which donates methyl groups to lower HCY and raise methionine, thus lowering your risk for developing a wide variety of diseases.

Choline has a number of crucial functions in the body and brain: it helps manufacture acetylcholine, one of the most important of the brain's chemical messengers. Deficiencies in choline can produce changes in mood, appetite, and behavior. In fact, choline treatment has been shown to bring about some improvement in people suffering from Alzheimer's disease. Choline also helps maintain the fluidity of cell membranes—remember, this is essential for health and vitality—and in one of its forms (*phosphatidylcholine*), it helps transport fats and cholesterol so that they can be either used by the body or "dumped." In fact, a number of studies show that fat and cholesterol are readily deposited in arteries and other tissues when choline is deficient. But when choline levels are sufficient, fat and cholesterol are transported via the bloodstream, then metabolized, excreted in the bile, or burned during exercise.

It is estimated that most of us get about 500 to 1,000 milligrams of choline per day from our food. Some good dietary sources of choline include beef liver, beefsteak, butter, cauliflower, coffee, eggs, iceberg lettuce, oranges, peanut butter, peanuts, potato, tomato, and whole-wheat bread. Some of these—especially cauliflower, iceberg lettuce, oranges, tomato, and whole-wheat bread—have additional dietary value as good low-fat, high-fiber foods.

Betaine: Betaine (also called *trimethylglycine,* or *TMG*) is actually a methylated version of *glycine,* our simplest amino acid. Betaine is a very efficient and direct dietary methyl donor, and it is a very effective treatment for extremely high HCY.

But betaine's health benefits can go much further than treating high HCY. Lab experiments with both rats and mice have shown that betaine greatly increases quantities of "good guy" SAM, and it does this at the expense of HCY. This means that betaine may help prevent and perhaps treat everything from heart disease and stroke to neurological diseases, psychiatric problems, and osteoporosis, in normal people. Some studies show that betaine greatly improves people's sense of well-being. In people with homocystinuria, betaine lowers HCY and greatly reduces the symptoms and progress of the disease. These symptoms and their by-products run the gamut from heart disease and stroke to mental retardation, neurological diseases, psychiatric problems, osteoporosis, and even dislocated eye lenses. It's also been shown, in rats, to reduce the accumulation of fats in the liver caused by alcohol consumption.

Betaine is found in many plants and animals and thus in many of our food sources. For example, there are large amounts of betaine in beets and spinach and probably in many other vegetables, but the amount varies. For example, the betaine content of spinach will vary depending on the salinity of the soil used to grow the spinach—something that you can't possibly know unless you're growing the spinach in your own garden.

Another plentiful source of betaine in the diet is seafood. While we have little information about the amounts of betaine found in most foods, vegetables and seafood are definitely on the recommended list—their betaine content is a happy bonus.

Methionine: Methionine is an essential amino acid and, as such, a vital component of proteins. Equally important, methionine is a pivotal part of methyl metabolism. We need methionine in methyl metabolism because it carries the methyl group in SAM. But methionine is a two-edged sword: it helps manufacture "bad guy" HCY, so too much methionine in the diet can be dangerous. In animal tests methionine caused severe clotting, blood circulation problems in the lungs, and even arteriosclerosis. In one study five of six rabbits were killed simply by giving them too much methionine.

We have a good idea of the general *range* of methionine that should be in the diet, but we don't know the optimal levels for maximum good health. Nor do we know what levels of other related nutrients, such as folic acid and choline, are optimal or how precisely these affect the optimal level of methionine. The dietary recommendations in this book are designed to provide an intermediate level of methionine that is not too far off optimal considering the other related components such as folic acid and choline.

Usually if people eat meat, fish, and/or dairy products three or four times a week, they already have reasonable levels of methionine. But there's good news for vegetarians: While not particularly rich in amino acids in general, some plant sources and combinations of plants can help keep methionine levels in a healthy range. Among the best of these are legumes, peanuts, and soybeans. Combine these with some grains such as brown rice and you'll be in pretty good shape. Vegetarians should use a combination of beans and whole grains to get a healthy amount of methionine.

THE METHYL MAGIC PROGRAM: FOOD ■ 51

Folic acid: Folic acid (sometimes called *folate*) is very important in methyl metabolism. A whole team or "corporation" of enzymes uses folate to help manufacture methyl groups from scratch.

You've probably read the latest research showing that folate is vital for preventing dangerous and even deadly birth defects known as *neural tube defects* (more about this in chapter 8). It also helps lower high levels of HCY. A number of studies have recently been published showing or indicating that folic acid levels higher than "normal" (the FDA recommends a daily intake of at least 400 micrograms) are important for maintaining low HCY, avoiding depression, minimizing DNA damage, and lowering risk of heart disease, stroke, and other vascular disease, as well as colon cancer.

But that's not all. Deficiencies in folic acid (it's one of the most common of all vitamin deficiencies) are associated with anemia (especially during pregnancy), cervical dysplasia, irritability, weakness, weight loss, apathy, anorexia, headache, heart palpitations, memory problems, hostility, paranoia, and digestive tract disturbances such as diarrhea. In fact, maintaining healthy levels of folic acid is considered so crucial that the Food and Drug Administration (FDA) has mandated that folic acid be added to all commercially sold enriched flour and other enriched grain products. This level is still quite low, though, so it's important to get even more folate from your diet and from supplements.

Folates are found in beans, orange juice (also oranges), green leafy vegetables, and many other foods. Besides green leafy vegetables like spinach, especially good sources of folates include organ meats, kidney beans, asparagus, broccoli, beets, yeast, cauliflower, cantaloupe, green peas, sweet potatoes, wheat germ, whole-grain cereals and breads, and lima beans. That's a wide variety of sources, and it's almost certain that even if you hate spinach, something on that list will appeal to your taste buds. At the same time, when you eat these foods, you'll be setting the stage for your own personal show of *Methyl Magic*.

Vitamin B$_6$: This essential vitamin actually is a family with at least three members: *pyridoxine, pyridoxal,* and *pyridoxamine.* No matter what the form, most of our body's vitamin B$_6$ is found in muscle, where it helps fuel the contractions that allow us to walk, run, jump, lift, and throw. It's also important as part of our defense against damaging free radicals—highly reactive oxygen molecules that can attack and alter or even kill cells. Vitamin B$_6$ helps convert the villain HCY into cysteine, which in turn helps fight off free radicals.

Vitamin B$_6$ is also a key player in methyl metabolism. It converts HCY to cysteine, thus lowering HCY and keeping it from inhibiting the transfer of methyl groups from SAM, an aspect of methyl metabolism. In combination with folic acid, vitamin B$_{12}$, zinc, and betaine, B$_6$ helps *remove* HCY, which in turn helps keep levels of methylation in the healthy range.

Because B$_6$ has many functions, a severe deficiency in the vitamin will cause a number of problems, including altered nervous function, seizures, dermatitis, inflammation of the tongue, cracked lips, carpal tunnel syndrome, and anemia. Clinical deficiencies in B$_6$ are rare, but subclinical deficiencies do occur in women and the elderly.

Also be aware that too much B$_6$ (more than 200 milligrams a day, especially taken alone and over a long time) can cause nervous system disorders. Chances are this is due at least in part to the fact that an overabundance of B$_6$ actually lowers methyl metabolism by converting too much HCY to cysteine instead of methionine. Remember that it's a combination of methylation of HCY and conversion of HCY to cysteine that keeps HCY levels in check, thus helping to prevent a Pandora's box full of diseases.

Vitamin B$_6$ is found in a wide variety of foods, especially poultry, fish, pork, bananas, and whole grains. So keep your cupboard and refrigerator stocked with these foods, and eat them on a regular basis. Watch out for pork, though, because it has a lot of saturated fats. Stick to the leanest possible cuts, or better yet, eat fish. These foods are yet another fundamental building block in your *Methyl Magic* program.

Vitamin B_{12}: Vitamin B_{12} (also known as *cobalamin*) is another key player in methyl metabolism. In combination with an enzyme and with methylfolate, B_{12} helps convert HCY to methionine, thereby helping to keep HCY levels in check. In addition, B_{12} lends a helping hand in the metabolism of carbohydrates, fats, and protein and also plays a role in the breakdown of amino acids and fatty acids. This versatile vitamin has a job in the brain as well: it helps manufacture many of the chemical messengers (neurotransmitters) that are so important in regulating our moods.

Early symptoms of serious B_{12} deficiency include dementia, poor attention span, and depression. If deficiency continues or gets worse, it can cause pernicious anemia, a potentially fatal disease of the blood, as well as potentially irreversible damage to the *myelin sheath* that insulates the spinal cord. Serious B_{12} deficiencies can also damage the brain, optic nerves, and peripheral nerves. This damage can ultimately bring on a condition called *subacute combined degeneration,* which can cause numbness, tingling, spastic paralysis, weakness, confusion, and depression. B_{12} deficiency occurs often in elderly people. Because B_{12} is inactivated by nitrous oxide—the "laughing gas" often used by dentists to kill pain—it's especially important that you take extra B_{12} after you've had this treatment.

Vitamin B_{12} is found in animals such as insects, meat, fish, and chicken. The list of good food sources of B_{12} is a long one: it includes organ meats like liver, kidney, and heart and seafood such as clams and oysters, which contain about 10 micrograms per 100 grams. Nonfat dry milk, crab, salmon, sardines, and egg yolk give 3 to 10 micrograms of B_{12} per 100 grams, while meat, lobster, scallops, flounder, swordfish, tuna, and fermented cheese contribute about 1 to 3 micrograms per 100-gram serving. B_{12} is found in smaller amounts in fermented soybean products, poultry, and fluid milk products.

Zinc: Zinc is an essential trace mineral, found in virtually all the tissues in the body—especially in the eye, kidney, brain, liver, muscle, and male reproductive organs, including sperm cells. Like vitamin B_{12}, zinc is an extremely versatile nutrient, playing pivotal roles in the activity of insulin, in the manufacture of proteins and DNA, and in healing wounds. Zinc also helps maintain bone structure, keeps the immune system peppy and on guard in the battle against disease, and even helps fight acne. In pregnant women, zinc helps keep baby's birth weight within a healthy range, thus reducing chances of illness and death in infants.

Zinc is also a star performer in *Methyl Magic*. The proteins that help turn genes on and off have appendages called *zinc fingers*, without which the turning on and off of genes can go dangerously awry. In fact, one of the most important enzymes in DNA regulation (DNA methyltransferase) is a zinc finger protein.

That's just part of zinc's role in *Methyl Magic*. Zinc also helps vitamin B_6 and enzymes keep levels of HCY in check by converting HCY to cysteine. Zinc also has an essential role in methylating HCY. The enzyme that uses betaine to make methionine by methylating HCY requires zinc to do its job.

Zinc deficiency can play havoc with our bodies. Too little zinc can create a "tired" immune system—and thus weakened defenses against disease. Zinc deficiency can also lead to sterility, lethargy, anemia, poor wound healing, skin inflammation, changes in hair and nails, dwarfism, and even loss of taste and smell.

In pregnant women, who are at high risk for zinc deficiency, low zinc can contribute to everything from extended pregnancy or prolonged labor to premature delivery or pregnancy-related toxemia, to retarded fetal growth and impaired development, which can include malformation of the brain and eyes, abnormalities of the heart, lung, skeleton, and genitals, and cleft palate. All in all, zinc deficiencies in the mother substantially raise the risk of infant mortality.

The best food sources of zinc are meat and seafood. This news may be upsetting to dedicated vegetarians, but plants, especially soy, generally don't have much zinc. Oysters, herring, milk, meat, and egg yolks are particularly abundant in zinc. Whole-grain breads and cereals do supply some zinc, but generally not the kind that is well absorbed by the body. In fact, the zinc in meat is four times as available to the body as that found in breads and cereals. Research has shown that as little as 3 ounces of beef a day (extra-lean, of course, to keep down your intake of saturated fats) can contribute significantly to maintaining healthy levels of zinc for efficient methylation.

Selenium: Selenium is an essential trace element with a chemistry similar to that of sulfur. It has many important tasks in the body, among the most vital of which is to serve as a powerful antioxidant. As such, selenium helps protect cells and the "energy factories" inside them from damage by free radicals. It also aids in fighting off poisoning from heavy metals such as mercury. In pregnant women selenium helps ensure normal fetal development. In addition, selenium is a vital aid in thyroid metabolism. There's also a growing amount of evidence that selenium can help prevent heart disease, control asthma, and stimulate the immune system. And keeping your body's selenium at healthy, moderate levels appears to be important in preventing cancer. Much evidence, both within the United States and worldwide, shows that cancer-related deaths increase when the selenium content in the soil, and thus local food and water, decreases.

Selenium is involved with methyl metabolism because of its functional forms. As the amino acids *selenocysteine* and *selenomethionine,* it can substitute in certain cases for the more common sulfur-based amino acids cysteine and methionine, which are needed to regulate HCY. In addition, some studies show that selenomethionine can raise the level of SAM in animals. Methylation also helps metabolize selenium so that it can be excreted in the urine, which is a good thing because too much inorganic selenium can contribute to heart and liver disease.

Foods likely rich in biological, organic selenium include broccoli, cabbage, mushrooms, celery, cucumbers, onions, garlic, radishes, brewer's yeast, grains, fish, and organ meats. These foods can still be low in selenium if they are grown on selenium-poor land. Generally selenium obtained through food is well absorbed by the body.

Inositol: This substance is an accessory to many of the methyl-boosting nutrients listed previously—especially folates, choline, vitamins B_6 and B_{12}, betaine, and methionine. Like choline, inositol helps mobilize fat, prevent unhealthy buildup of fats in the liver, and maintain our cell membranes.

Good food sources of inositol include some fruits, especially oranges, grapefruit, and grapefruit juices, cantaloupe, and limes. Stone-ground whole-wheat bread, cooked beans, and green beans also supply inositol.

CONCLUSION

Think of your *Methyl Magic* program as a house under construction. In the chapter you've laid the dietary foundation for your house in the form of a generally healthy diet, and you've begun to build the walls by focusing on the foods that contain ingredients—choline, folic acid, and the rest—that will boost your methyl metabolism and keep it running smoothly. But you've still got less than half a house. In the next chapter you'll get the detailed blueprints for finishing off your construction project, the final keys to preventing a wide variety of diseases, for maintaining your body and mind in a state of energetic good health, and perhaps for extending your life. Houses, after all, especially well-built, solid ones, can resist storm and flood and often last more than a hundred years.

CHAPTER 5

THE METHYL MAGIC
PROGRAM: SUPPLEMENTS

Learning without thought is labor lost;
Thought without learning is perilous.
—*Confucius*

In the last chapter you've built the foundation of your *Methyl Magic* house, and you've made a good start on building the walls. But to have a good, solid edifice to keep your methyl metabolism in good tune, to finish off the house, you'll need to get those walls all the way up and get a roof over your head. To do that, you'll need more help than you can get from food alone. You'll need to use dietary supplements, specific supplements specially selected for their methyl-boosting properties. I can't state this strongly enough: *It's impossible to perform* Methyl Magic *using food alone. You* must *augment your diet with methyl-boosting supplements.*

You've no doubt heard, perhaps from your doctor or from health columns in newspapers or magazines, that "we get all the vitamins we need from our food." This is often stated as if it were a scientific fact. Well, it's not a fact, and it's not very scientific. Actually, it's an example of a little knowledge, just half the story, being dangerous. It's a myth born of the misapplication of science.

The truth is that humans evolved to derive necessary nutrients from eating a variety of foods from nature. This variety of food contains a range of proteins, carbohydrates, fats, vitamins, and minerals, from which most of us get the nutrients we need. After all, we've been doing this for millions of years, so we know it must work. Yes, it works; on that most everyone agrees. But what does it work *for*?

Remember, we *evolved* to be able to derive necessary nutrients from our food. Evolution works by making animals that are good at reproducing. But most animals—ourselves included—are designed to reproduce when we're young, usually *very* young. For all but the last fifty or so years of our several-million-year evolution we didn't first go to college or plan our financial strategy for retirement before starting a family. So in general we evolved to get all the vitamins we need from our food *for the sake of reproducing when young.*

But when we talk about what we need, are we talking only about what we need for youthful reproduction? When you talk with your doctor about what to do to ensure good health, is your only concern with reproducing? Remember, most of us have our children when we're in our teens, twenties, and thirties. That's less than half our lives. What about the rest of our lives, while we're raising our children and after our children have gone on to have children of their own? Most of us would like to stay healthy and avoid disease as long as we can—not just during our reproductive years, but throughout our lives. In other words, we need healthful longevity.

Well, unfortunately evolution doesn't guarantee us healthful longevity. Relying on a variety of foods from nature, or from the grocery store, doesn't guarantee us healthful longevity, either. Now, it's true that we are beginning to understand some of the nutritional factors we need to maintain our health and extend our longevity. But this new understanding still doesn't amount to a guarantee.

Boosting methyl metabolism isn't necessarily a guarantee that we'll all enjoy a long and healthy life, although more and more evidence points in that direction. For example, a number of studies suggest strongly that we should lower our levels of HCY to help prevent not only high levels of HCY, but also heart disease and some types of cancer, and perhaps even to slow down the aging process. We can't accomplish this entirely through diet alone; we have to use dietary supplements. The most generally effective means to boost methylation—thus lowering levels of HCY and raising levels of "good guy" SAM—is through a combination of supplements listed in this chapter. In addition, this chapter gives you a number of alternate plans for taking these supplements— just pick the plan that best suits your taste, your schedule, and your lifestyle.

Here's a specific list of supplements for methyl metabolism. Taken daily, these are designed to provide nutritional support against the diseases, both physical and psychological, that can make your life miserable if your methylation machinery has gone awry. In most cases a range of doses is given to make it easier to find the appropriate tablets.

Betaine (also called trimethylglycine, or TMG): 750 to 1,000 milligrams a day. Anhydrous betaine or betaine monohydrate are generally available as powders, and this is a convenient form to take. Anhydrous betaine provides about 15 percent more betaine per gram, but that's not a significant difference. Betaine powder is very soluble in water, juice, and the like. I usually put it in water or juice, but I have also put betaine in coffee, tea, soy milk, soft drinks, even beer and wine! But remember that betaine tends to absorb water from the air, so keep jars of betaine well closed. Otherwise it will become slushy and unpalatable. This doesn't happen, even over years, if betaine is stored in sealed containers such as jars or quality Ziploc bags. Betaine is also available in tablet form.

Choline: 250 to 500 milligrams a day. Choline is usually available in tablets as choline bitartrate or in liquid as choline chloride solution. Either form is perfectly acceptable. If you don't take betaine, then amounts of choline between 750 and 1,500 milligrams should assure a good supply of methyl groups for methyl metabolism. Build up to this dosage gradually, however. Taking 1,500 milligrams of choline at once without working up to it will make some people hyperactive, anxious, or both. So start with 250 milligrams choline a day and over a month or so increase as desired to the 750- and 1,500-milligram level. Generally younger people are more likely to respond to choline, so people in their thirties and younger may want to increase the dosage more slowly and use a low level of choline supplementation—say, 250 to 750 milligrams. As we get older our uptake of choline, at least into the brain, appears to be less efficient, and higher levels may be useful, such as 750 to 1,500 milligrams. Some people complain that choline supplements cause a fishy odor. I have never encountered a fishy smell with choline as long as I take it with folic acid, as in the combined formulas that follow.

Folic Acid: 800 micrograms a day, either as a specific tablet or as part of a multivitamin tablet. Folic acid is a perfect example of a methyl-boosting nutrient that's far more effective as a supplement than when taken only through food sources. The body does a better job of absorbing folic acid from supplements than from food. In addition, if foods are cooked excessively, there's a risk of losing the folic acid.

Keep in mind that folic acid is somewhat sensitive to heat and should be stored in the refrigerator.

Some people avoid taking folic acid supplements because they've heard—or have even been told by their doctors—that folic acid can be toxic. All of us—especially pregnant women and heart patients—do ourselves a disservice if we let this advice sway us. The truth is that in *very rare* instances folic acid can be toxic, but only if taken *in large amounts* (over 1 milligram), and only if taken *without vitamin*

B_{12}. Note: Folic acid may be partially inactivated if taken at the same time as either vitamin C or iron.

Vitamin B_{12}: 250 to 500 micrograms a day, in the form of sublingual tablets. It's important to keep in mind that folic acid and B_{12} work together. A good rule of thumb is that folic acid and B_{12} should always be taken together, either at the same time or on the same day.

Vitamin B_6: 20 to 50 milligrams a day, either as a specific tablet or as part of a multivitamin formula.*

Zinc: 20 to 50 milligrams a day, either as a specific tablet or as part of a multivitamin formula.*

Vitamin E: 400 to 800 International Units (IU). Vitamin E isn't mentioned in the food chapter for a very good reason: it's virtually impossible to get optimal amounts of this crucial nutrient from food alone. Current Recommended Daily Allowances range from 4.5 to 18 IUs, which many experts agree is far less than what's needed for optimal health.

Vitamin E is a powerful agent in sustaining health and preventing disease. Mountains of scientific studies over the years have revealed vitamin E's amazing versatility. For example, vitamin E protects polyunsaturated fats from destruction by free radicals. We need polyunsaturated fats to maintain the health of our cell membranes, nerves, and vascular systems, as well as for the synthesis of powerful local hormones called prostaglandins, which are vital to the proper functioning of our hearts and kidneys. Vitamin E is also a potent antioxidant and an immune system booster. There are

*These nutrients can be found in the specified amounts in many multivitamin preparations. Again, check the label. For pregnant women, multivitamins should also contain a full 800 micrograms of folic acid.

also reports claiming a role for vitamin E in preventing cancer, including breast cancer, and in reducing fibrocystic breast disease and the symptoms of premenstrual syndrome (PMS).

There are four variants of the vitamin E molecule, which is known scientifically as *tocopherol*. The four varieties are *alpha, beta, gamma,* and *delta tocopherol*. Get a natural vitamin E product (they come in gel capsules, tablets, and powders) that contains a mixture of all four tocopherols. The label on the bottle should tell you—it should name all four, or read "natural, mixed tocopherols."

Note that only alpha tocopherol supplies officially recognized vitamin E activity. However, recent evidence shows that the other tocopherols, especially gamma, can do some antioxidant or free radical scavenging jobs better than alpha. So a formula containing 300 to 600 milligrams of mixed tocopherols, with all four tocopherols (alpha, beta, gamma, and delta) listed, is also a good choice.

While vitamin E is not a methyl supplement per se, it does affect some of the same aspects of health related to proper methylation. For example, vitamin E is important for stabilizing the healthy essential oils that can improve methyl metabolism.

A note of caution: People who take anticoagulation drugs, who have reduced coagulation factors or vitamin K deficiencies, should know that vitamin E might make their conditions worse. These people should discuss their vitamin E requirements with their doctors. The same may be true for some cancer patients, so they should consult with their doctors before taking vitamin E supplements.

Vitamin E is somewhat sensitive to heat and oxygen, so it's best to store it in your refrigerator. Vitamin E may be inactivated by iron, so it is best to take it separately from any iron supplements.

Fish oil: 600 to 1,200 milligrams a day. If you're not eating fish two to three times a week, you'll need to take fish oil supplements. Fish oils have been shown to lower HCY levels. Fish oils contain polyunsaturated fatty acids—especially the omega-3 fatty acids *EPA* (*eicosopentaenoic acid*) and *DHA* (*docosahexaenoic acid*)—that we need to help protect our cell membranes, nerves, and vascular systems, and to aid in the synthesis of prostaglandins. Fish oils may also be useful in treating arthritis and other inflammatory disorders, including psoriasis.

The fish oils recommended here are fish body oils, *not* fish liver oils. Look for the following on the label: each 1,000 to 1,200 milligrams of fish oil should contain about 160 to 350 milligrams of EPA and 100 to 150 milligrams of DHA.

(Caution: In diabetics fish oil is reported to increase blood sugar and decrease insulin secretion. Diabetics should not use fish oil supplements without being advised to do so by their doctor. Also, people predisposed to bleeding or hemorrhaging should use fish oil supplements only if advised to do so by their doctor.)

Inositol: 250 to 500 milligrams a day. Inositol is a sugar that the body uses to package fats and also to send chemical signals from one part of a cell to another. It's convenient to think of inositol as a partner of choline: both are important components of the cell membranes in the brain, central nervous system, muscles, and other tissues; and the body uses both to help package and mobilize fatty acids and cholesterol. In fact, most choline sold in the health food store contains equal amounts of inositol. There are no official recommended daily intakes or any recognized toxicity for inositol. I usually recommend that people take 250 milligrams of inositol mainly as balance for choline supplements. Inositol is reported to have some benefits similar to those of choline, and inositol and choline are often combined in supplements. So if your choline supplement contains 250 milligrams of inositol, you won't need extra amounts of the latter. Again, check the label.

Selenium: 50 to 200 micrograms a day.* While selenium is essential, some forms of selenium, such as sodium selenate, can be toxic in large amounts. Therefore, specific recommendations here are for moderate supplements of selenium preferably in one of two forms: either selenomethionine or yeast selenium.

Methionine: Not recommended. Although some scientists and doctors think of methionine as a methyl supplement, methionine by itself is usually not a good choice. Usually if people eat meat, fish, and/or dairy products three or four times a week, they already have adequate levels of methionine. In fact, people often have too much methionine compared to the folic acid, betaine, and other factors in their diets. If your HCY is elevated, it may simply be a matter of too much methionine in your diet. So obviously you don't want to make things worse by taking methionine supplements.

The first four recommended supplements—betaine, choline, folic acid, and vitamin B_{12}—are best taken in the morning. They can be taken with or without a meal. If you're taking betaine hydrochloride, do so with a substantial meal. This form tends to generate an excess of stomach acid and thus indigestion. These nutrients can be taken without having to change the foods you eat, but it always helps to lay the good dietary foundation described in the previous chapter.

*These nutrients can be found in the specified amounts in many multivitamin preparations. Again, check the label. For pregnant women, multivitamins should also contain a full 800 micrograms of folic acid.

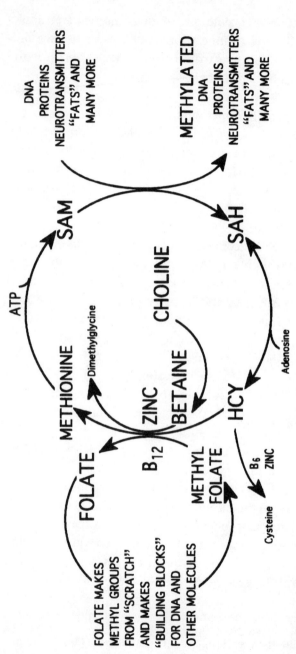

Methyl Metabolism

Here's the big picture! Refer back now and then as you need to through the rest of the book. Adapted from Cooney, C. A. (1993). Are somatic cells inherently deficient in methylation metabolism? A proposed mechanism for DNA methylation loss, senescence and aging. Growth, Development & Aging 57, 261–73.

Examples of four supplementation programs are given so that you will have a formula to use even if one component, such as betaine, is not available in your local health food store. If you prefer to take fewer tablets per day, consider examples C and D. The best, most complete supplementation program is given in example A; B is preferable to C; and C is preferable to D.

SAMPLE PROGRAMS

Example A

Betaine powder, tablets, or capsules: 750 to 1,000 mg a day

Choline and inositol tablets: 1 daily tablet containing 250 mg of each nutrient

Folic acid: 1 daily tablet containing 800 mcg (or a 400-mcg tablet plus 400 mcg from your multivitamin)

Vitamin B_{12}: 1 daily sublingual tablet containing 500 mcg

Vitamin E: 1 daily gel cap or tablet containing 400 international units (IU) in a natural, mixed-tocopherol form (or as an alternative, a formula containing 300–600 mg mixed tocopherols)

Daily multivitamin and multimineral tablet(s) or capsule(s) with a standard recommended dose that contains 20–50 mg zinc, 20–50 mg vitamin B_6, and 50–200 mcg selenium (some as L-selenomethionine)

Fish oil: 1–2 daily gel caps totaling up to 1,000 mg

Example B

Choline and inositol: 1 daily tablet containing 250 mg of each nutrient; work up to 1,000 mg*

*Gradually, over one month, increase the choline to 1,000 mg. For example, take 250 mg choline each day for the first week, 500 mg each day for the second week, 750 mg the third week, and 1,000 mg from then on. It's okay if the inositol goes up at the same time or if you leave it at 250 mg. This is the same as Example A, except that it substitutes choline for betaine. Your metabolism will produce betaine from some of this choline.

Folic acid: 1 daily tablet containing 800 mcg or a 400-mcg tablet plus 400 mcg from your multivitamin

Vitamin B_{12}: 1 daily sublingual tablet containing 500 mcg

Vitamin E: 1 daily gel cap or tablet containing 400 IU in a natural, mixed-tocopherol form

Fish oil: 1–2 daily gel caps totaling up to 1,000 mg

Daily multivitamin and multimineral tablet(s) or capsule(s) with a standard recommended dose that contains 20–50 mg zinc; 20–50 mg vitamin B_6, and 50–200 mcg selenium (some as L-selenomethionine)

If you don't like taking pills or powders in the quantities in Examples A and B, here are two examples of supplementary strategies to cut down the intake and still get most of the methyl-boosting nutrients you need:

Example C (Minimalist Formula 1)

Betaine powder, tablets, or capsules: 750 to 1,000 mg a day

Choline and inositol tablets: 1 daily tablet containing 250 mg of each nutrient

Vitamin B_{12}: 1 daily sublingual tablet containing 500 mcg

Daily multivitamin and multimineral tablet(s) or capsule(s) that include in the dose recommended on the bottle the following:

Folic acid: 400–800 mcg a day

Vitamin E: 200–800 IU a day (preferably natural)

Zinc: 15–50 mg a day

Vitamin B_6: 20–50 mg a day

Selenium: 50–200 mcg (some as L-selenomethionine) a day

In this example the polyunsaturated fatty acids of fish oil will have to come from your foods and your metabolism.

Example D (Minimalist Formula 2)

Folic acid: 1 daily tablet containing 400 mcg

Vitamin B_{12}: 1 daily sublingual tablet containing 500 mcg

Vitamin E: 1 daily gel cap or tablet containing 400–800 IU in a natural, mixed-tocopherol form

Daily multivitamin and multimineral tablet(s) or capsule(s) with a standard recommended dose that contains 20–50 mg zinc, 20–50 mg vitamin B_6, and 50–200 mcg selenium (some as L-selenomethionine)

If you don't like taking tablets, there are liquid or powdered vitamin formulas that are acceptable substitutes. Choline, for example, is available in liquid formulas, while betaine is available as a water-soluble powder. It's not physically possible to get all of the previously outlined recommended nutrition in a single tablet that anyone smaller than a horse could swallow, so it's best to take a combination of several tablets or use liquid formulas.

While there are many brands of vitamins, I like the quality and purity of products from Nature's Plus, Nature's Way, Twinlab, and the Life Extension Foundation. If these brands aren't available at your local health food dealer, you can find the companies by calling the toll-free directory service (1-800-555-1212). If you have a computer and access to the Internet, you can find them by searching the World Wide Web. Also see appendix III.

YOUR DOCTOR'S ROLE

These dietary recommendations are intended for normal healthy adults as a form of nutritional insurance. People with serious health problems can work with their doctors to design an overall nutrition and health program consistent with their particular treatment and needs.

There are some treatments for several diseases in which methyl supplementation as previously described may be incompatible or pose other risks. The first of these is cancer. While there is evidence to suggest that methyl supplementation will help prevent cancer, we don't know what methyl supplementation will do in people who already have cancer. It may or may not be beneficial. So until it is tested it is not recommended.

There are times when people should not take methyl supplements without good medical supervision and medical approval. Generally if you are under a doctor's care or wish to treat a disease, you *must* consult your physician and/or psychiatrist before starting any significant supplement or nutrition program—including *Methyl Magic*. This helps your doctor provide you with the best treatment and to understand or prevent any confounding factors in your treatment.

Some drugs and conditions are, or may be, incompatible with methyl supplements. The following is a known list of these:

Manic depression: Although folic acid has been used in conjunction with the antipsychotic drug lithium to treat manic depression, methyl supplements are not necessarily recommended for manic depression because they may actually trigger a "switch" from depression to mania. So methyl supplements might be useful for the treatment of manic depression but would need to be managed carefully under medical and psychiatric supervision.

Insomnia: In general, methyl supplements tend to increase alertness and wake you up when you may want to sleep. So it's a good idea to take methyl supplements in the morning rather than at night. People who already have trouble sleeping should consider this before taking supplements and should consult with their doctors.

Anxiety: If you tend to be chronically anxious, or have been diagnosed with general anxiety disorder, SAM might make you even more so. This is the one downside of this otherwise "good guy." So methyl supplements that boost production of SAM may not be a good idea. Again, if you have this existing condition, you should consult with your doctor before taking *Methyl Magic* supplements.

Parkinson's disease: The effects of *Methyl Magic* supplements on this disease are not clear. On the one hand, Parkinson's, a nervous system disorder, can be complicated by the increased breakdown and excretion of dopamine in the brain via methylation by SAM. If you break down too much dopamine, it can cause depression and bring on or worsen Parkinson's-like symptoms. (One of the causes of Parkinson's is a shortage of dopamine.) Many people who suffer from Parkinson's are treated with the drug L-dopa, which stimulates the brain's production of dopamine. Where L-dopa is used to treat Parkinson's disease, drugs that inhibit L-dopa methylation and breakdown in the blood are often given in tandem. However, some research suggests that reduced rates of methylation may actually be implicated in the disease itself. Again, *ask your doctor.*

Epilepsy, seizures, and convulsions: Many antiepileptic and anticonvulsive drugs may act in part through inhibiting some methylation reactions or methyl metabolism in general. Some research indicates that methyl supplements could make these conditions worse or interfere with treatment. On the other hand, some evidence suggests that improving methylation might help prevent some seizures. This is clearly an area where more research is needed. In particular, women with epilepsy who want to bear children need an effective treatment for their disease but at the same time want to prevent birth defects. Again, you should *ask your doctor* before taking *Methyl Magic* supplements.

Methyl Magic is based on data from the leading scientific and medical journals with which your doctor should be familiar. So take this book along the next time you pay your doctor a visit. Besides protecting your health, another reason to work with your doctor on your nutrition and treatment is that a number of tests, including HCY and other measures relating to your health, can be made before and during the time you go on your *Methyl Magic* program. This way you and your doctor can monitor your levels of HCY to determine if your methyl-boosting supplements and foods are doing their job. My guess is that if you follow the *Methyl Magic* program diligently, you and your doctor will be pleasantly surprised.

CHAPTER 6

THE METHYL MAGIC PROGRAM: EXERCISE

I n any program designed to improve your health and prevent disease, diet and exercise should go hand in hand. *Methyl Magic* is no exception. While methyl-boosting nutritional supplements remain the key to this program, you'll be doing yourself and your methyl metabolism a great favor if you get out and exercise.

Why? It has to do with our now familiar villain: HCY. In general, moderate excercise is associated with lower HCY levels. The Hordaland study in Norway, for example, found that for most people—especially those in their sixties and older—HCY levels went down as physical activity went up. It's also been shown in scientific tests that the lower your body mass index (BMI), the lower your HCY levels, and vice versa. The best and most reliable way to reduce your BMI is through a combination of diet and exercise.*

However, during the Boston Marathon some runners experienced as much as a 40 percent reduction in levels of choline. Remember that choline is essential to methyl metabolism. The message here is that if you're exercising in a reg-

---

*To calculate your BMI, divide your weight in kilograms by the square of your height in meters. Alternatively, multiply your weight in pounds by 703, then divide by the square of your height in inches. While the guidelines change from time to time, for most adults a BMI between 20 and 25 is considered healthy. If your BMI is over 25, health risks, especially the risk of high HCY levels, increase.

ular and highly strenuous way, you need to take methyl supplements—especially choline—to replace what you've depleted during exercise.

There are other reasons why exercise and *Methyl Magic* go together. It's important to exercise to improve circulation, which in turn helps mobilize HCY to be processed; its accumulation would play havoc with your health. Improving your circulation also helps mobilize nutrients—including methylating nutrients—so that your cells can use them.

If your goal is to lose weight, it's probably important to combine exercise and methyl supplements along with a healthy diet. Methylation is a key to moving fat, while excercise is a key to burning it off.

The goal is to exercise enough (thirty minutes or more at a time) to elevate your heart rate, break a good sweat, and stimulate blood flow and circulation throughout your body—especially in the peripheral blood vessels that feed your extremities. This will help keep blood levels of HCY in the normal range. Activities in which you alternately dilate and constrict your peripheral blood vessels should help accomplish this. Doing aerobic exercise—jogging, walking, cycling, and most sports—for thirty minutes three times a week should do the trick. To augment the methyl-boosting effects of exercise, try a sauna and massage, both of which improve blood circulation.

If you prefer anaerobic exercise such as weight lifting or other forms of strength training and bodybuilding, you'll want to pay special attention to this cautionary note. Many weight lifters eat a high-protein diet or take protein powders in the belief that this helps build muscle. Unfortunately, high levels of dietary protein—for example, any amino acid–balanced protein mix—will also contain a significant amount of methionine, which is likely to raise levels of HCY. Thus, it's especially important that you also take methyl-boosting supplements, which contain enough folic acid, vitamin B_{12}, vitamin B_6, and methyl donors betaine and choline to help process the extra HCY. After all, rippling muscles are no guarantee of clear arteries.

My own experience is a good testimonial for the partnership of diet, methylation supplements, and exercise. Before I started my own *Methyl Magic* program, my physical stamina was poor, and I was experiencing chronic pain in my joints. Since I was a dedicated racquetball player (I now cycle and play golf), it goes without saying that these problems were taking the joy out of an activity I dearly loved and that should have been helping to keep me healthy.

But once I started methylating, both these problems virtually disappeared. The pain in my joints receded to the vanishing point, while my stamina increased tremendously. Now, several years later, I can enjoy exercise and have the energy and tirelessness of a man twenty years younger.

So be sure to make regular, moderate exercise a part of your *Methyl Magic* program. Walk, hike, run, play tennis or golf, ski, or just get out in the garden and move some dirt around. In tandem with your diet and supplement program, exercise will keep your HCY levels down, probably raise your levels of "good guy" SAM, and help you reap all the rewards of a methylated life.

CHAPTER 7

ALCOHOL, SMOKING, AND METHYLATION

We've all heard about the potential health hazards of drinking and smoking: liver, heart, and lung disease, respiratory problems, and so on. But alcohol and tobacco also have adverse effects on methylation.

ALCOHOL

When you drink alcohol, you're walking a tightrope. Drink too much over a long period of time, and you'll fall off the rope on the side of diminished methyl metabolism. Drink too little or not at all, and you'll fall off on the other side, losing the proven health benefits of moderate drinking.

Since this book is about methylation, let's start on that side of the rope. Along with the other health dangers of excessive drinking (increased risk of colon cancer, liver disease, and psychiatric and nervous system disorders), alcohol has long been known to compromise methyl metabolism. In particular, alcohol is known to adversely affect the metabolism of folate. Here's how: Once in the body, alcohol is converted first to acetaldehyde, then, in a second step, to acetic acid—in other words, vinegar. It's the first step, the conversion to acetaldehyde, that causes the problem, because acetaldehyde depletes methylfolate. That's the very form of folate the body needs to remethylate HCY, thus keeping levels of HCY in the healthy range.

Actually, the relationship between alcohol and methyl metabolism is complex. On the one hand, as we've already seen, alcohol use in excess compromises aspects of methyl metabolism that use folic acid and vitamin B_{12}. At the same time, however, alcohol can have a beneficial effect on methyl metabolism. That's because alcohol enhances the transfer of methyl groups from betaine to HCY to make methionine—the very process that helps keep HCY levels in check. So if you're taking betaine as one of your Methyl Magic supplements, this may decrease some of the adverse effects of alcohol on methyl metabolism.

There are even strong indications that methylating supplements can be used to treat some of the ravages of alcoholism. One of the hazards of excessive alcohol in the body is that it causes the unhealthy accumulation of fats in the liver. This fatty accumulation is an early stage in alcoholic liver injury. It's also been shown that cirrhosis of the liver inhibits the activity of methylating enzymes that make beneficial SAM, among other methylators.

But there's more to this story. For example, scientists have already shown that in baboons "good guy" SAM reduces liver injury due to alcohol. At the Veterans Affairs Medical Center in Omaha, Nebraska, a team led by Dr. Anthony Barak has studied rats, looking at betaine as an alternative source of methyl groups when the folate B_{12} pathways are compromised by alcohol. Even in perfectly sober rats, the scientists found that dietary betaine can more than double the amounts of both betaine and SAM in the liver. In alcoholic rats, liver betaine and SAM are reduced compared with the levels in sober rats. But when these alcoholic rats are given betaine along with their booze, the levels of both betaine and SAM rise above normal. In fact, levels of SAM in the liver can rise to six times the normal amounts! This means increased methyl metabolism, which in turn may render at least some protection against damage due to excessive drinking.

The relationship between methylation and alcohol doesn't stop here. Among its numerous functions, the liver packages fats as triglycerides. High liver trigyceride levels have been associated with liver disease. Dr. Barak and his colleagues showed that while alcoholic rats accumulated about six times the triglycerides in their livers as did the controls, betaine could protect the rats from most of this dangerous accumulation. In fact, alcoholic rats fed betaine had less than twice the accumulated liver triglycerides as their cousins who received no betaine and no alcohol. As a bonus, the betaine also protected the rats from alcohol-induced weight loss. In fact, one scientist holds two patents for the use of betaine to treat a hangover. The effective levels of betaine used in these rat studies were about 300 milligrams per day (a high dose for a 200-gram rat!). The levels of betaine for protection of humans from alcoholic fatty liver have yet to be determined.

Do different varieties of alcohol have differing effects on methylation? Maybe. Grape juice is known to have significant amounts of choline, so it may be that the alcoholic version of grape juice—wine—is also rich in either betaine or choline. We know very little about the betaine or choline content of other varieties of alcohol, but we do know that alcohol itself stimulates the body's use of betaine, which in turn helps produce "good guy" SAM.

There's even more evidence that alcohol consumption and methylation are related. In a recent study published in the *Journal of the American Medical Association,* Dr. Eric Rimm of the Harvard School of Public Health in Boston and co-workers looked at over eighty thousand women over fourteen years in the Nurses Health Study. They showed that women with the highest folate intakes (over 400 micrograms per day from food and supplements) and who had about two drinks a day suffered only 22 percent as many coronary heart attacks as did women who had the lowest folate intakes and were non-drinkers. Neither drinking nor high folate alone produced anywhere near this reduction in heart attack. The following figure, using data from Rimm's study, shows that a high folate intake (more than 400 micrograms a day) combined with two drinks a day reduces the risk of heart attack to only 22 percent that of women with low folate intake who don't drink.

Rimm, et al., divided alcohol consumption into three categories: nondrinkers, those who consume 0.1 to 14.9 grams of alcohol per day, and those who consume 15 or more grams of alcohol per day. Using these amounts, one drink would equal

4 ounces wine (½ cup), 14 g alcohol

8 ounces beer (1 cup), 14 g alcohol

1 ounce whiskey (2 T), 14 g alcohol

Two drinks would be the equivalent of

8 ounces wine (1 cup), 28 g alcohol

16 ounces beer (2 cups), 28 g alcohol

2 ounces whiskey (4 T), 28 g alcohol

Note: Alcoholic beverages vary in their alcohol content, so the above is only a general guideline.

In this study—as with so many others—generally the highest folate intakes were due to vitamin supplements and/or fortified breakfast cereals. This suggests that a daily folate supplement of 800 micrograms is a good way to reduce the risk of a heart attack. These researchers also showed that women with the higher B_6 intakes (more than 3 milligrams per day) had the lowest risk of heart attack. This study and others show a huge reduction in the occurrence of heart attacks with methyl-boosting supplements. Imagine if these levels of reduction could be achieved nationwide. Heart attacks would probably no longer be our major killer and might not even be a worry for most people!

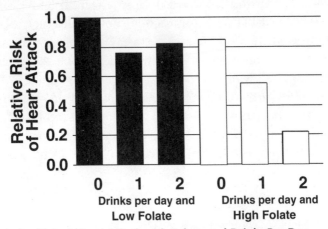

Relative Risk of Heart Attack with Folate and Drinks Per Day

Rimm, et al., demonstrated that increased folate intake reduces the risk of heart attack. In particular, the highest levels of folate (>400 mcg/day) combined with two drinks per day reduces the risk of heart attack to only 22 percent of the risk faced by women with low folate intake who don't drink. Adapted from Rimm, E.B., Willett, W.C., Hu, F.B., Sampson, L., Colditz, G.A., Manson, J.E., Hennekens, C., Stampfer, M.J. (1998). Folate and vitamin B$_6$ from diet and supplements in relation to risk of coronary heart disease among women. *JAMA* 279, 359–64.

One note from my personal experience: When I first started taking methyl supplements I couldn't drink any more than half a beer without getting a headache within about half an hour. After a couple of months this effect largely went away. No one else has reported this effect to me, even if I told them ahead of time, so this may just be my particular genetics. But if it does happen to you, and the effect returns every time you drink over the course of a month or more, you might want to see your doctor for advice.

Warning: The contents of this chapter should not be interpreted to mean that you can drink all you want and still avoid the ravages of excess simply by taking methylating supplements. Also, drinking can lead to alcoholism and isn't for everyone. I'm only recommending that if people drink, they may have a greater need to take methyl supplements than do nondrinkers. But I'm not recommending total abstinence from alcohol, either. Too many studies show health benefits from moderate drinking—less stress, less cardiovascular disease—to ring the chimes of prohibition. In sum, I want to encourage people to drink only in moderation to take advantage of these health benefits and especially to keep their methyl metabolism in tune. One to two drinks a day, particularly of red wine, should confer those benefits and keep people from falling off the tightrope in either direction.

SMOKING

Aside from playing catch with hand grenades or swimming with sharks, smoking is probably one of the worst things you can do for your health. Smoking's role in bringing on cancer and heart disease is well-known. But relatively few people know that smoking has an adverse effect on methylation. In humans smoking raises HCY and depletes folates. One study reports that in the lungs of guinea pigs, nicotine reduces both SAM and its metabolite SAH. Reduced SAM and SAH suggests that methylation is being compromised. These may constitute some of the underlying reasons that smokers have a much higher risk of developing cancer and heart disease.

So my advice here is simple. Advice 1: Don't start! Advice 2: If you've already started, quit! That way you'll help ensure that your methyl metabolism won't be compromised and thus decrease your risk of developing serious diseases.

CHAPTER 8

FOR WOMEN ONLY

Nature has cast a kind eye on women in a number of ways. Women tend to live longer than men; they have a higher percentage of body fat and thus are better protected against cold weather; they have lower rates of heart disease and some forms of cancer; and they're better at making lasting social bonds that help enrich and even insure their lives. It's not really surprising that these things are true—women carry and to a large extent raise our young, especially in vulnerable infancy, so evolution has a vested interest in granting them special protection.

Nature has offered women the same kindness in regard to methyl metabolism. They're simply better at it than men. This is especially true of young women, who are in the prime of their childbearing years. I sometimes think that women have better methyl metabolism than men because women take a much greater interest in food, nutrition, and supplements than do men. In my experience there are probably ten women who take a real interest in methylation and other kinds of supplementation for every one man who does. This seems ironic, because in some respects men are in greater physiological need of appropriate nutrition and supplements to help prevent heart disease; yet men seem to have less interest. Even female rats are more resistant to methyl deficiency than are male rats. Methyl-deficient diets will readily cause cancer in male rats but apparently not in female rats.

Other studies show that estrogen is clearly a factor in improving methyl metabolism in rats.

Women are also at an advantage in regard to DNA methylation. Why? Basically because women have two X-chromosomes—one of the biological "cradles" that contain all our genes—while men have only one. What does this have to do with methylation? DNA methylation inactivates one of the two X-chromosomes, so that some cells have one version, or *allele,* of the X-chromosome genes active, and other cells have the other alleles active. So even if a woman has an X-chromosome mutation, about half her cells will still express the "normal" X-chromosome. You could think of this as nature having a choice of X-chromosomes and hedging its bets so that women effectively use some genes from each chromosome. Men, on the other hand, have only one X-chromosome. If it's defective, a man's got no backup, no insurance policy from nature. That's why women are largely unaffected by X-linked diseases like hemophilia A or Menkes disease that might very seriously affect men.

But none of this makes women—even lady rats—immune to methyl deficiency and its related diseases. For example, even though their rates of heart disease may be lower than those of men (women's HCY is lower than men of the same age, probably thanks to the action of estrogens and related "female" hormones), women are still much more likely to die of heart ailments than of breast cancer. This may be the result at least in part of a slowdown in their methyl metabolism—the result, for example, of a shortage of vitamin B_{12}—which in turn increases their levels of "bad guy" homocysteine.

So for this and many other reasons—some of which we'll discuss in a moment—women need *Methyl Magic* as much as, and perhaps even more than, men. To maintain efficient methyl metabolism, then, women need to follow the diet and supplement program outlined in this and previous chapters.

This is especially true at two of the most important junctures in a woman's life: pregnancy and menopause. Let's start with pregnancy. A growing baby—and, for that matter, a nursing baby—make heavy nutritional demands, often at the expense of mom. During pregnancy (in lab animals) the body's levels of methyl-boosting nutrients choline and betaine are diminished in the mother when compared with levels in nonpregnant females. These nutritional shortfalls can bring on a host of problems during pregnancy, both for mom and for her burgeoning baby. Let's first have a look at the dangers that poor nutrition in general—and sagging methylation rates in particular—can present to mom.

ANEMIA

Pregnant women are especially vulnerable to a blood disease known as *megaloblastic anemia,* in which the red blood cells accumulate too much hemoglobin and swell beyond their normal size. Hints that the disease are present include paleness and general weakness. If untreated, it can lead to disturbances in the gastrointestinal or nervous systems. In fact, it was while doing research on megaloblastic anemia in the twenties and thirties that Lucy Wills discovered women with anemia could be cured when given a preparation of yeast.

The significant ingredient in the yeast preparation, known for some time as the "Wills factor," was eventually identified as folic acid, the important methyl-boosting supplement described in earlier chapters. And to the great good fortune of pregnant women everywhere, folic acid was eventually shown to both prevent and treat megaloblastic anemia.

A shortage in the intake or absorption of vitamin B_{12} can cause basically identical symptoms as folic acid deficiency. So it's important to take both folic acid and B_{12} to help avoid anemia. It's also important when having your blood tested to check levels of folate, vitamin B_{12}, MMA, and HCY.

PREECLAMPSIA

Preeclampsia is a disease of pregnancy, the symptoms of which include high blood pressure, excessive weight gain, water retention, severe headache, and visual disturbances. If left untreated, preeclampsia can lead to full-blown eclampsia, which can bring on convulsions and even coma. In 1995 scientists discovered that high levels of HCY is a risk factor for preeclampsia: 101 patients with a history of severe early-onset preeclampsia were tested at least ten weeks postpartum for high HCY. In this study 14 of 79 patients tested did indeed have elevated levels of HCY. The researchers recommended that women with a history of preeclampsia be screened for HCY to avoid recurrence of the disease in future pregnancies.

CHOLESTASIS

Cholestasis of pregnancy is caused by a blockage of bile flow from the liver. Signs are itching, dark urine, pale stools, and, in some cases, jaundice. Some experts think that cholestasis may be the culprit in many cases of otherwise unexplained stillbirths.

The disease has been treated successfully with SAM. This makes it likely, although not certain, that methyl supplements—which, as you recall, help boost production of SAM—would help prevent cholestasis or treat it when it does occur.

RHEUMATOID ARTHRITIS

Occasionally symptoms of rheumatoid arthritis—a disease in which cells from one's own immune system attack tissues in the joints, causing pain, swelling, and inflammation—appear in women during or just after pregnancy. Some researchers have linked rheumatoid arthritis with deficits in methylation and essential fatty acids. So methyl-boosting supplements may help keep this painful disease at bay.

MULTIPLE SCLEROSIS

This disease—often called simply MS—is caused by destruction of the myelin sheath, which wraps around and insulates the nerves. Women with MS will sometimes show an increase in symptoms just after pregnancy. As we said before, pregnancy and nursing put enormous demands on mother's metabolism and nutrient supplies. Although MS is a distinct disease from methyl deficiency, MS has many symptoms very similar to vitamin B_{12} or folic acid deficiency. Methylation and healthy oils and fats are needed for myelin sheath repair as well as for maintaining a healthy immune system, both important in MS. A *Methyl Magic* program may help in prevention of, and recovery from, this sometimes devastating disease.

POSTPARTUM DEPRESSION

The period just after pregnancy is over—and sometimes pregnancy itself—is often lowlighted by feelings of deep depression. While it's not yet been shown scientifically that pregnancy-related depression is linked with sagging methylation rates, research has revealed time and time again that garden-variety depression and poor methylation often go hand in hand. So it's at least an educated guess that declines in methylation rates are also implicated in depression that comes during or after pregnancy. Just one more reason for pregnant women to start and maintain a *Methyl Magic* program.

HEALTHY BABY

Pregnant women need to keep their methylation rates at optimal levels not only to protect themselves, but to help ensure the health of their babies. (This is especially true during the first month of pregnancy, but it's also true throughout pregnancy and during the nursing period.) Perhaps the most worrisome danger is the now well-established link between low methylation rates and birth defects. Of these, among the most common—and devastating—are neural tube defects (NTDs), a group of spinal conditions that can leave baby deformed, paralyzed, or even dead. Neural tube defects include a broad spectrum of gruesome cranial, spinal, and nervous system malformations, including *anencephaly*, in which a large part of the baby's brain is missing (these babies almost always die in infancy), *encephalocele,* a sort of hernia of the brain, and *spina bifida*. In its most severe form, this defect leaves part of the baby's spinal cord, as well as some of its nerves, lying outside the vertebrae in the back, vertebrae that normally protect these vital nervous system connections. The results can be paralysis and, in a small percentage of cases, death.

The NTD story features as villain our now familiar bad guy, HCY. As I mentioned earlier, pregnant women normally have the lowest levels of HCY in any adult population group. But if HCY levels are high during pregnancy, owing to genetic and/or dietary deficiency of methylating nutrients, there is a strong risk of NTDs.

No prospective mother wants to deal with the horrors of neural tube defects. Luckily there's an easy fix, and it has to do with keeping up those methylation rates. For pregnant women, taking folic acid—either alone, with vitamin B_{12}, or as part of a broad supplementation program of the *Methyl Magic* variety—will usually do the trick, helping to prevent these awful and life-threatening conditions. And you don't have to be already pregnant to start taking them. Many experts, including Dr. Godfrey Oakley of the Centers for Disease Control in Atlanta, emphasize that it's important for *all* women of childbearing age to take folic acid or a prenatal supplement with folic acid. The reason for this is that damage to the fetus occurs before many women even know they're pregnant. Dr. Oakley even gives bottles of folic acid tablets as wedding presents!

Even though there's little doubt that folic acid (and B_{12}) supplementation can prevent NTDs, there's still some controversy concerning the proper amounts. The level of folic acid in enriched grain products as of 1998 is still quite modest, so a multivitamin or individual folic acid and vitamin B_{12} supplements are still a good idea. I recommend at least 800 micrograms of folic acid and 250 to 500 micrograms of vitamin B_{12} a day. This will cut the risk of spina bifida by half or more. Recent research in rats and mice suggests that inositol may prevent some of the NTDs that escape folic acid supplementation.

NTDs are not the only danger to pregnant women whose methylation rates are low. If HCY is high (remember, high HCY is an indication of subpar methylation rates), the risk of early miscarriage is much greater. But in studies where women had a first, or more than one, pregnancy resulting in an NTD baby or in early miscarriage, folic acid treatment—and the resulting decline in HCY levels—led in nearly all cases to subsequently successful and healthy pregnancies for mom and baby.

It's a good idea for any woman entering her childbearing years—whether she's already pregnant or not—to have her HCY checked. This simple blood test is described in chapter 3 and can be done through your doctor's office. If HCY is high even with daily doses of folic acid (800 micrograms) and B_{12} (500 micrograms), along with other good nutrition, then there are other measures that can correct this.

These measures, worked out with your doctor,* could include increased folic acid (4 micrograms per day) or betaine (3 grams per day). But for the vast majority of women, the levels of nutrients recommended in this book should be adequate to control HCY.

CHOLINE IN EMBRYONIC AND NEWBORN DEVELOPMENT

Folic acid and vitamin B_{12} are by no means the only methyl-boosting substances that affect the health and well-being of your baby. Newborns require large amounts of choline for growth. In humans, as well as in other animals, much of the needed choline comes from mother's milk; however, this can leave a new mother with choline deficits. In animal experiments, scientists have found that the amount of choline in breast milk generally coincided with the amount in the mother's diet. So it's important for nursing mothers to keep up their dietary intake of choline. There's another good reason to watch your choline intake. Experiments in lab animals have shown that babies whose mothers were given supplemental choline during pregnancy had better memories than those whose mothers received no supplemental choline. Supplementing mothers with choline produced memory improvement that lasted for the offsprings' entire lives. In fact, these offspring did not show the old-age-related memory loss seen in "normal" old animals.

To help prevent the many problems just listed, and to reap the rewards of improved methylation, pregnant women

* A woman taking anticonvulsants (antiepileptics) such as diphenyl-hydantoin, phenobarbital, valproic acid, or carbamezapine must consult with her physician prior to taking folic acid supplementation or other "methyl" supplementation. Folic acid and some other supplements may interfere with the action or effectiveness of these anticonvulsants.

need a *Methyl Magic* program designed especially for them. The following is a conservative version of such a program, but even this should be done under a doctor's supervision:

A CONSERVATIVE *METHYL MAGIC* PRENATAL PROGRAM

A daily prenatal multivitamin containing:
> Folic acid: 800 mcg
> Zinc: 20 to 50 mg
> Vitamin B_6: 10 to 25 mg
> Selenium (some as L-selenomethionine): 50 to 200 mcg

Choline and inositol tablets (daily): Start with 1 tablet per day containing 250 mg each of choline and inositol, then after a few weeks add a second tablet; the total should be 500 mg each of choline and inositol

Vitamin B_{12} (daily): 1 sublingual tablet containing 250 to 500 mcg

Vitamin E (daily): 1 gel cap or tablet containing 400 IU in a natural, mixed-tocopherol form

Fish oil (daily): 1 to 2 gel caps totaling 1,000 to 1,200 mg

BEYOND BABIES

Just because your last child has finally entered kindergarten—or college, for that matter—your need to keep your methyl machinery in good order doesn't stop. For women throughout life, and especially during and after menopause, it's vitally important to stick with the *Methyl Magic* program. For if your methylation rates fall, which they almost certainly will as you get older, you'll be leaving yourself vulnerable to a number of nasty diseases.

Anemia: Low levels of methylating nutrients folate and vitamin B_{12} have long been associated with anemia. In fact, when doctors see women with anemia, especially in its more severe forms, they immediately look for B_{12} or folate deficiency. Ask your doctor to check your iron, B_{12}, folate, and HCY when you have a blood test. Low iron can also be a cause of anemia but should not be considered the sole cause without thorough tests. And remember, iron supplements alone will not cure a folate or B_{12} deficiency. Still, until menopause it's not a bad idea for women to take multivitamins that contain B_{12}, folic acid, and iron. After menopause the need for iron diminishes, so postmenopausal women might be wise to switch to an iron-free multivitamin.

PMS: Numerous studies indicate that vitamin B_6 as well as other nutrients (including magnesium, zinc, and essential fatty acids, and generally multivitamins and minerals) are of help in lessening the severity of premenstrual syndrome (PMS). Although the role of methylation in PMS has yet to be determined, the fact that methylating supplements can help relieve symptoms (in particular, B_6 is reported to help relieve depression, irritability, and fatigue) is a strong indication that methylation rates may decline just before or during PMS. Certainly a good nutritional program, including at least moderate supplements of these and other nutrients as recommended in this book, is worth trying.

Note that high levels of B_6 supplementation (over 200 milligrams a day), especially taken alone and over a long time, can cause nervous system disorders. This is probably due at least in part to diversion of HCY away from methyl metabolism. So keep your B_6 supplementation at about 25 to 50 milligrams a day, and be sure to also supplement with folic acid and vitamin B_{12}.

Cervical dysplasia: Cervical dysplasia is a change in the state of cells in the cervix. It can, but doesn't always, lead to cervical cancer. Here again, methylation may play an important role. If a woman is infected with a bug known as *human pa-*

pillomavirus (HPV-16), or if she has other risk factors for cervical dysplasia (use of oral contraceptives is one example), low levels of folate in her red blood cells can heighten the risk, whereas high levels of folate can diminish risk. One side note: Studies that investigated invasive cervical cancer risk did not show a correlation between low folate and actual cervical cancer. It's still not a bad idea to take folate supplements as an insurance policy.

Depression: Women are three times more likely to suffer from depression than are men. Curiously, despite better methyl metabolism in many respects—reflected in generally lower levels of HCY—women also have lower blood levels of "good guy" SAM than men. In fact, some studies show that women's blood levels of SAM are as much as 30 percent lower than men's. Low blood SAM is strongly correlated with, and is probably a cause of, depression.

Scientists have used folic acid and other methyl supplements—including SAM itself—to effectively treat depression in both women and men. Because depression is at least sometimes caused by poor nutrition and because poor nutrition will not be corrected by antidepressant drugs, good nutrition with an emphasis on methyl supplements is an important part of avoiding depression or minimizing it when it does occur. This is increasingly important with age, because the occurrence of depression and the rising levels of HCY that contribute to it both increase as we get older. We'll go into this in greater detail in chapters 14 and 15. For now, just keep in mind that *Methyl Magic* can help prevent depression and can be an important, even necessary, part of helping to treat the disorder.

Lupus: Lupus is one of the so-called autoimmune diseases, in which your immune system attacks your own body, subjecting it, as it were, to "friendly fire." Women are about ten times as likely as men to develop this disease. The consequences can be grave indeed: inflammation and scarring of the skin, and kidney damage leading to protein depletion. Examinations of lupus patients have shown, among other changes, that the T-cells in these patients' immune systems have lower levels of DNA methylation than do T-cells of healthy controls. Recently it's been shown that folate deficiency in women can cause declines in methylation of immune system cells called *lymphocytes*, among which are the T-cells. T-cells, then, may well be losing DNA methylation, so it seems prudent to maintain a healthy diet with a focus on methylating supplements to help maintain DNA methylation of lymphocytes.

This is especially true because of the apparent link between lupus and heart disease. A 1997 study compared over a thousand women with lupus to an equal number of women who were not afflicted with the disease. The study revealed that women with lupus in the thirty-three to forty-four age group were over fifty times more likely to have heart attacks than their peers who did not have lupus. Because methyl deficiency and high HCY are risk factors for heart disease, it's especially important for women with lupus to pay attention to their nutrition, again focusing on methylating supplements—with your doctor's approval and advice, of course.

Oral contraceptives: Are you on the Pill? Well, it may surprise and disturb you to know that the Pill may be taxing your methyl metabolism. In fact, use of oral contraceptives (OC) has long been associated with lower levels of vitamin B_6 and a higher incidence of vascular disease. More recent studies confirm that lower levels of folates, vitamin B_{12}, and vitamin B_6 are found in women using OCs. Again, it pays to have your doctor check your levels of HCY. If they're high, then that's a risk factor for heart disease, especially in women on the Pill.

Menopause and after: One of the unfortunate hallmarks of aging in women (and men, too) is an inexorable rise in HCY levels. A large Norwegian study, the Hordaland Homocysteine Study, showed that women in their early forties had an average HCY level of 9.1 micromolar. Women in their mid-sixties, however, had HCY levels of 11 micromolar, an increase of more than 22 percent.

Some researchers have claimed that HCY rises as a specific aspect of menopause, but others see this as part of the general rise that occurs with age. In either case, by now you know that HCY can nearly always be lowered with methyl-boosting supplements.

It's known that *hormone replacement therapy* (*HRT*), usually with a combination of estrogen and progesterone, lowers HCY in postmenopausal women. In fact, a recent Dutch study showed that one variety of progesterone reduced HCY levels by as much as 16.9 percent. (Another recent study shows that estrogen even lowers HCY in elderly men!) But don't rely on HRT entirely without also maintaining good dietary habits and a careful program of methyl supplementation.

Osteoporosis: Although scientists do not yet consider the case closed, many—myself included—think that rising levels of HCY with age contribute to the development of *osteoporosis,* the "brittle bone" disease that plagues so many women in their later years. One tantalizing piece of evidence is that osteoporosis is usually found in people with homocystinuria (remember, that's the disease marked by abnormally high levels of HCY), even when they're only a few years old. So it's definitely worth considering as another possible advantage of keeping HCY low via methyl-boosting supplements.

That doesn't mean you should throw away your calcium and magnesium, though. It's a good idea to keep up your calcium intake and to include a multimineral and multivitamin pill that has at least the RDA of vitamin D and magnesium. Estrogen replacement therapy, which helps prevent osteoporosis, has also been shown to lower HCY levels.

Heart disease: Some of the same deficiencies in methylating nutrients that can lead to heart disease in men can also affect women. A huge study of over eighty thousand women by Drs. Eric Rimm, Meir Stampfer, and their colleagues at the Harvard School of Public Health in Boston revealed that women who had low intakes of folate and vitamin B_6 had significantly higher risk for heart disease than women who took in an average of 400 to 1,000 micrograms of folate and about 6 milligrams of vitamin B_6 a day. (The most popular sources for these *Methyl Magic* nutrients were multivitamin supplements.) "Intake of folate and vitamin B_6 above the current Recommended Daily Allowance," the researchers concluded, "may be important in the primary prevention of coronary heart disease among women."

CONCLUSION

Women have as much to gain from a *Methyl Magic* program as men, perhaps even more. Not only can methyl-boosting supplementation lower the risk of heart attack, anemia, depression, and the like, it can also help make for a trouble-free pregnancy, help prevent birth defects, and perhaps soften the impact of PMS.

CHAPTER 9

LIFE AND METHYL POWER

The simple, bedrock truth is, *without methylation there could be no life as we know it*. Even before we're conceived, methylation influences the genes that come from our mothers and fathers, the genes that ultimately make us what we are—different from everyone else on the planet. Once the explosion of conception takes place, methylation is critical in guiding the development of the embryo and to assigning an almost infinite variety of job descriptions to each of the cells in our bodies. Methylation is a crucial feature of our nervous systems, enabling the metabolism of chemical messengers (neurotransmitters) in the brain and body and maintaining the nerves themselves in good working order. In other words, methylation affects how we feel and how we think. Methylation helps regulate the production of melatonin, the hormone that helps regulate our internal biological clocks, so it's even one of the determining factors in when and how well we sleep.

This is the most technical chapter of *Methyl Magic* and talks about cellular and molecular events common to most of our cells and tissues. If you instead prefer discussions of how *Methyl Magic* can help prevent heart disease, cancer, and other diseases you can skip ahead to chapter 10.

Affecting how we think and feel as well as when we sleep are all high-profile tasks, biological versions of glamour jobs. But methylation's widely varied role in maintaining life and health includes a number of jobs that, though less glamorous, are equally vital. One of these is the regulation of fluidity in the "walls," or *membranes*, that surround our cells. You may recall that this fluidity keeps the important chemicals—sodium, potassium, and many others—flowing in and out of cells at proper, healthy rates.

Here's how this works. Our cell membranes are made up of a double layer of lipids ("oily" fats connected to water-soluble molecules) that act as insulation of the fluids inside our cells against fluids from the "outside"—for example, blood plasma or cerebrospinal fluid. It may help to think of this insulation as a wall, with "gates," "tunnels," and "bridges" that serve as checkpoints for incoming and outgoing chemical traffic. Using a combination of proteins, enzymes, and electrical signaling, the "wall" keeps this traffic flowing smoothly and helps ensure that the "city"—the cell itself—is neither under- nor overpopulated and is in chemical balance with its surroundings.

This insulation is essential to life, to the functions and regulation of cells. Within the cell membranes themselves, the "building blocks," as it were, of the cell "walls" are a great number of proteins. These proteins can act as enzymes, facilitating chemical reactions in the cells; as receptors, providing a "dock" where incoming substances can "put in" to the cell; or as transport proteins, giving life's substances a "ride" from one place in the cell to another.

These membrane proteins communicate with the outside by receiving and sending signals, in the form of hormones, and they maintain the cell by importing and exporting materials—calcium, magnesium, and amino acids, as well as sodium and potassium. The activity of these proteins in the membrane depends on how fluid the membrane is. Methylation makes cell membranes more fluid—it's as simple as that. Cholesterol, by the way, makes cell membranes less fluid.

You might want to imagine this fluidity as the difference between a lake filled with water and a lake filled with molasses. Imagine trying to play water polo in each of these lakes. The players in the molasses lake would have difficulty making their passes, swimming toward the goal, even playing the game at all. It's the same with the proteins in your cell membranes: the thickness of the medium can make a big difference in the ability of the proteins to move around and do their jobs.

A number of studies have shown that membrane fluidity decreases with aging. These changes in membrane fluidity can have significant effects on membrane protein function, cellular signaling, and so forth. The membrane fluidity may be part and parcel of the general slowdown of body mechanics that seems to be an inevitable feature of growing older.

You'd think there would be little we can do to affect a microscopic and highly complex process like cell membrane fluidity. Well, look again. Methylation of fatty substances known as *phospholipids* in the cell membranes generally increases membrane fluidity. How can we enhance this methylation? There are a number of ways. One is by adding SAM to cells. In general, boosting methyl metabolism (and/or reducing HCY) by means of *Methyl Magic* supplementation may also help maintain methylation of membrane phospholipids and membrane fluidity.

Methylation also has important roles in the disposition of fat in our bodies. It's clear that methylation mobilizes fat, much in the same way it increases the fluidity of cell membranes. In particular, methylation helps move fat out of the liver, where it will accumulate if you are methyl deficient. You don't want to suffer the consequences of that fatty accumulation, because it can be a prelude to either liver cancer or cirrhosis, both potential killers. Luckily SAM, betaine, and choline have been shown to mobilize fat in the liver and get it into the bloodstream and bile. From there the excess fat can be burned by the muscles and otherwise "flushed" from the body. This fat mobilization also helps keep fats and cholesterol from settling in other body tissues—especially the blood vessel walls, where it can contribute to heart disease and stroke.

Because methylation is so basic, nature provides us with not one, but two distinct pathways to convert HCY to methionine—the fundamental conversion that keeps methyl metabolism humming along in a healthy way. In one of these pathways, various versions of folic acid make methyl groups. With the help of various enzymes, these folates (versions of folic acid) produce methyl groups from other simple molecules like carbon dioxide. With the help of vitamin B_{12} and enzymes, folates methylate HCY and convert it to methionine. Each molecule of folate and each molecule of B_{12} can perform these reactions over and over again.

In the other pathway, betaine donates a methyl group to HCY to make methionine. However, in the process, betaine gets consumed. This is why it takes small, milligram, amounts of folic acid but larger, gram, amounts of betaine to reduce HCY in the blood plasma.

Methionine, an essential amino acid derived from the foods we eat, is also an essential aid to methyl metabolism. There are several ways in which methionine renders invaluable assistance. First of all, it acts as a methyl donor in some of the same ways betaine donates methyl groups. Methionine also acts as a team player with other substances to carry methyl groups from one molecule to another—in some ways the same kind of team play we find between folate and vitamin B_{12}. Methionine and HCY (the latter can be seen simply as demethylated methionine), along with SAM and SAH, signal the status of methyl metabolism to various enzymes in our cells. This signaling in turn helps regulate methyl metabolism, keeping it from slowing down or "misfiring" and thus protecting us from a broad spectrum of diseases.

DNA METHYLATION

The human genome—the "dictionary" of genes that make us what we are—contains three billion building blocks, or "letters." These building blocks are known as *bases*. Actually there are only four types of bases, or "letters," in the DNA "alphabet": adenine, cytosine, guanine, and thymine, usually abbreviated A, C, G, and T. All these bases fit into the nucleus of a single human cell, something you can't even see without a microscope. These bases are organized into twenty-three chromosomes (including X and Y "sex" chromosomes), which in turn contain an estimated total of about one hundred thousand genes. Actually, in most of our cells we have two copies of all of the above genes, one copy from each parent. So that makes a grand total of six billion bases, organized into forty-six chromosomes, including two X chromosomes if you're a woman, or including an X and a Y chromosome if you're a man.

Even at this tiny molecular scale, if these chromosomes were unraveled and the DNA stretched end to end, the DNA from just a single cell would be two meters long. Some scientists have estimated that if the human genome were printed on regular pages in a typical type font, these pages would make a stack as high as the Washington Monument! Think of a human being as a scaled-down version of this enormous book. How does such a book—a human being—get organized?

Once a sperm cell penetrates an egg and the little explosion known as conception takes place, the new embryo—later, if all goes well, to be a new baby—is little more than a few cells. These cells don't really have much by way of an identity, except for a job description that tells them whether they're going to be liver cells, lung cells, or skin cells. How do those cells get their identities? In large part from DNA methylation.

Keep in mind that DNA is put together in basically the

same way in most of the cells in our bodies. So how is it that we have thousands of different types of cells that make up our internal organs, our skin, our eyes? The difference in your various cells is in the genes that they express. Your liver expresses somewhat different genes and makes a somewhat different set of proteins and enzymes than your skin or your brain. In other words, those differences in gene expression define each of our cell types and differentiate them from one another.

What regulates the expression of genes that ultimately defines the varied tasks of our bodies' cells? DNA methylation. How? By shutting down the expression of genes that the particular cell type doesn't need. The genes are still there—they've just been silenced. Early in the development of an embryo, when there are relatively few cells and very few cell types, DNA methylation determines what types of cells— lung, liver, skin, and so on—these cells will become as they divide and multiply. So DNA methylation is absolutely essential for the embryo to develop into a functioning, healthy human being. In fact, it's been shown in laboratory mice that without DNA methylation embryos can't survive. This means that for us, *without DNA methylation life comes to a screeching halt.*

But what happens if cells get "amnesia," causing them to lose their memory of what type of cells they are and what jobs they're designed to do? If that happens, cells may lose their ability to pass on to their "offspring" cells information about their identities and duties. In adults this cellular "amnesia" could contribute to autoimmune diseases or ailments in which organs fail to function properly. For example, this "cellular amnesia" could help instigate the development of some types of diabetes. Worse yet, some of our previously normal cells may become cancerous cells. Some experts believe that this sort of "cell amnesia" is part and parcel of the aging process. So obviously this "cellular amnesia" can play havoc with our health and in the end even kill us.

So how do we keep our cells from developing this potentially life-threatening "amnesia"? That's where DNA methylation comes in. DNA methylation is one of the fundamental ways that gene expression is controlled, so that cell types remain strictly defined and remember their identities. After all, we wouldn't want a skin cell to reproduce itself as a liver cell. The fact that every cell in our bodies has at least a slightly different methylation pattern than every other cell makes the task of DNA methylation even more difficult and complex.

Basically that task is executed by an enzyme known as *DNA methyltransferase, (DNA MTase* for short). There may be more than one of these enzymes, but so far only DNA MTase has been well characterized. DNA MTase picks up methyl groups from SAM and transfers them to molecules of DNA. DNA MTase also binds zinc, which appears to help DNA MTase function, although we don't yet know exactly how.

But DNA MTase does more than just transfer methyl groups from SAM. It also maintains the pattern of DNA methylation from one cell generation to the next. It's a form of "biological photocopying": the enzyme copies methylation patterns from one strand of DNA to the other strand. Thus, when DNA has just replicated and has one old, parental strand and one new, daughter strand, the DNA MTase can copy the parental methylation pattern onto the daughter strand. This process is called *maintenance methylation.* Like other methylation, life can't go on without it.

How do we know all this? Well, a number of experiments with plants show that changes in DNA methylation will cause big changes in the size, height, and leaf and flower structure of the plants. In mice, researchers have looked at mutations in which a type of gene known as a *repetitive jumping gene* has "hijacked" control of another gene that determines the color of the mouse's coat. So instead of having a normal, dark (black to brown) coat, this jumping gene makes the mouse yellow. But these jumping genes don't always perform their color conversion trick well. In fact, most of these mice whose genes tell them to be yellow are only partially yellow, and some don't look yellow at all! What keeps these jumping genes in line? In large part it's DNA methylation, acting like a policeman to at least partially silence the expression of the renegade jumping gene. This "disciplinary action" carried out by DNA methylation not only returns the mice partly or fully to their original dark coat color, it also makes them healthier. The black or brown mice are leaner and have less cancer and diabetes than their yellow siblings.

Recently we have used yellow mice to show that feeding methyl supplements to pregnant female mice produced more dark-coated and fewer yellow-coated offspring. Although we are not yet sure, chances are that DNA methylation is involved in this phenomenon. We also showed that healthy, dark-coated mothers produce more healthy, dark-coated offspring even without supplements. This means that the effects of methyl supplements may carry through to the next generation of offspring. In other words, diet and methyl supplements may have cumulative effects on health and longevity over several generations.

The jumping gene that created the strains of yellow mice is actually one of a class of genes known as *endogenous retroviruses* (*ERVs*). In mice these ERVs can cause problems far more serious than a change in coat color—cancer being one example. These ERVs and similar genes are found not only in mice, but in humans. Their expression has been linked to a number of nasty ailments: Sjögren's syndrome, an autoimmune disease that dries out the mucous membranes in the eyes and mouth; Graves' disease (characterized by an overactive thyroid gland); and at least one form of immune system deficiency known as CD4+ T-cell immunodeficiency. ERVs also bear some similarities to the AIDS virus. One of these ERVs, known as *human endogenous retrovirus* (*HERV*), has been associated with a variety of human diseases, including systemic lupus erythematosus, rheumatoid arthritis, insulin-dependent diabetes mellitus (IDDM), some connective tissue diseases, psoriasis, and a number of inflammatory diseases of the nervous system. So without DNA methylation to "police" these ERVs, these diseases and others would almost certainly strike us at far greater rates.

DNA methylation may also play a role in human cancer, the number two cause of death in America. That's because DNA methylation has much to do with keeping chromosomes, and the stuff they're made of (chromatin), together, organized, and properly condensed. A large body of scientific evidence shows that drugs or diseases that partially block DNA methylation will cause chromosomes to break, unwind, and decondense. Such treatments, especially those using a powerful DNA methylation inhibitor called *5-azacytidine*, will also cause gain or loss of chromosomes in cells. Many of these chromosome breaks and unravelings are of the same type that occur as cancers develop.

We need DNA methylation to keep our chromosomes intact and organized. So that's a very good reason—a whole list of good reasons, actually—to start your *Methyl Magic* program. By doing so, you'll give your body the components to keep your DNA methylation machinery in good tune and thus give yourself a running head start on preventing one or all of these debilitating ailments.

METHYLATION, LIFE, AND GENETIC SCIENCE

Two types of genetic studies show how important methylation is to life. The first type, done in mice, are known collectively as "knockout" studies. The second are natural, rare types of inborn genetic errors of methyl metabolism in humans.

KNOCKOUT MICE

In mice you can precisely "knockout" a gene by engineering a very similar, but defective, gene, then adding it in the laboratory to special cells taken from mouse embryos very early in their development. Once these special, very early embryonic cells, called *embryonic stem (ES)* cells, have the modified gene, they are returned to early-stage mouse embryos. With the help of these surrogate embryos and a surrogate mother mouse, scientists can use the same batch of modified cells to make several baby mice.

Some of these baby mice will now have the new "knockout" gene in their *germ line*—their sperm or eggs. (Sometimes mice of two different coat colors are used so that researchers can see which baby mice have more cells with the engineered gene.) Once you have at least one mouse with the knockout gene in its germ line, you can breed it to produce mice that reliably have one copy of the knockout gene. You can also breed these mice so that they have two copies of the knockout gene. Animals with one copy of a given knockout gene are called *heterozygotes*, while those with two copies of the knockout gene are known as *homozygotes*.

When scientists first made the gene that knocked out the DNA MTase enzyme, the early embryonic cells into which the knockout genes were implanted seemed fine. So did the mice that ultimately developed from these genetically altered cells. When the researchers bred the heterozygote mice with each other, the rules of genetics dictated that a quarter of the baby mice should have been homozygotes. But *none* of the babies were homozygotes. That was the first tip-off that something strange was going on.

The second tip-off came when the scientists went back to look at the homozygote embryos. They found that a number of those embryos were retarded in development: many of them were missing visible forelimb buds and had underdeveloped organs and more cell death than normal embryos. These genetically altered homozygote embryos stopped developing after eight to eleven days (normal gestation in mice is twenty-one days). This experiment showed that DNA methylation, or at least the DNA MTase gene, was essential for mouse embryos to develop into healthy mice. Presumably this gene is also essential for embryonic development of other mammals, including humans.

This knockout gene experiment was one way of demonstrating that DNA methylation was critical in the lives of mice and probably of humans as well. A second demonstration focused on a protein that has a "preference" for latching onto methylated DNA. This is part of the machinery that makes DNA methylation work. This protein was investigated for its biological role by inactivating the gene that constituted the protein's "blueprint." When researchers inactivated this gene, they found that ES cells could still survive. But for some reason, when the scientists tried to grow male mice from these male ES cells, the mice had severe developmental defects. This proved that yet another step involved in control of the genome by DNA methylation is essential for development and normal life.

Eventually scientists found that what was critical for genes involved in DNA methylation was also vital for genes that regulate other kinds of methylation. There are probably at least one hundred types of genes that are blueprints for methylating enzymes found in both mice and men. In an experiment with one of these enzymes, Dr. Steven Clarke and his co-workers at UCLA and UC San Francisco knocked out the gene for an MTase that works in partnership with SAM to repair certain types of protein damage that occur with age. This MTase is found in organisms ranging from simple bacteria and yeast to far more complex organisms—mice and humans, for example.

When Dr. Clarke and his team first made heterozygote mice who still had one good copy of the MTase gene for this protein repair enzyme, these mice were fine. When the scientists bred their first homozygous mice, these also seemed healthy in most ways, except that they grew just a bit slowly. Remember that because both copies of the gene had been knocked out, these mice apparently had almost none of the protein repair enzyme—it measured at less than 1 percent the amount of a normal mouse. Even though the deficiency didn't seem to trouble the mice much early in their lives, it eventually showed up in the most dramatic way possible, and drastically shortened their life span. Normal mice live an average of two years, but the mice lacking the protein repair enzyme gene lived an average of only forty-two days.

At first these early deaths were a mystery, because when they did autopsies on the dead mice Dr. Clarke's team couldn't find anything that could have killed the animals. So the scientists set up videocameras to observe the remaining mice while they were still alive. The videos revealed that the mice had severe seizures. Often these seizures were fatal. The scientists eventually found that several tissues of these knockout mice had dangerously low rates of protein repair. This was particularly true in the brain—thus the seizures and the dramatically shortened life spans. So here was yet another form of methylation that was, and is, crucial to a normal life.

Of the roughly fifty types of MTase enzymes found in both mice and humans, so far only these two have been the focus of "knockout" experiments like those previously described. Obviously both aspects of methylation are vital to a long and healthy life. It wouldn't be surprising if most, if not all, aspects of methylation will eventually be found to be as crucial to life as these two.

HUMAN STUDIES

Studies in mice are always interesting, in that mice in many ways are similar to humans. But they're not identical, so to get a clearer picture of methylation it's important to look at human studies. One of the ways scientists first learned about the importance of methyl metabolism in human health was through people who had inborn errors of metabolism—that is, genetic defects in their ability to metabolize certain components of their food, such as the amino acid methionine. One of the results of these inborn errors can be homocystinuria, which was one of the first clues to the importance of methylation in human life. To refresh your memory, homocystinuria is a rare genetic disease that results in very high levels of HCY in the blood and in the urine. (People with homocystinuria have blood levels of HCY ten to one hundred times higher than those in most people.) Homocystinuria can result from a severe methyl deficiency. Afflicted patients often suffer from poor mental development as well as other seriously abnormal features.

Homocystinuria is actually a group of diseases in which any of several of the critical enzymes or transport proteins connected with methyl metabolism can be defective. In our chromosomes we have a gene for each of these enzymes and proteins from our mother and father. Anyone who inherits just one defective copy of any of these genes may have hyperhomocysteinemia—moderately elevated HCY—and be at great risk for developing life-threatening and debilitating disease in the long term. But those unfortunate enough to inherit two defective copies, one from each parent, will usually have homocystinuria and develop life-threatening and debilitating disease from early childhood.

People with homocystinuria appear to develop normally in the womb, presumably because they can rely on mother's methyl metabolism. Once they are born and metabolically "on their own," though, problems start to arise. Beginning in infancy, homocystinurics can develop a variety of serious, often life-threatening, disorders, including

- mental retardation
- arteriosclerosis
- dangerous blood clots, which can lead to heart attacks and strokes
- detached optic lenses
- osteoporosis
- abnormal glucose tolerance
- elevated plasma insulin
- sleep apnea, a dangerous interruption or cessation of breathing during sleep
- psychiatric disorders, especially depression
- seizures
- gait disturbances

Mental retardation occurs in a majority of homocystinurics, with the average IQ less than 70. While mental retardation is not reversible, it is apparently preventable by early diagnosis and treatment. Many of the other effects listed are also preventable by early intervention, and several effects are reversible later in life. If begun early enough in life, lowering HCY can partially relieve, or even prevent, mental retardation.

Homocystinuria is treatable for two main reasons. First, some patients have less severe enzyme defects than others. If the defects are mild enough, they can be overcome by supplying large amounts of the specific vitamin needed to boost activity of the defective enzyme. The second reason is more complex. Two metabolic pathways exist in normal people that allow HCY levels to be lowered by converting HCY to methionine. One of these pathways uses folic acid to make the necessary conversion. If the folic acid pathway is defective, another enzyme that uses betaine as a source of methyl groups can convert HCY to methionine. If the body gets enough betaine, this "substitute" pathway will take over the job, helping reduce HCY to near normal levels.

Fortunately nearly all homocystinurics respond to one form or another of treatment that usually includes betaine and large doses of either folic acid, vitamin B_6, vitamin B_{12}, or some combination of two or more of these methylating nutrients. Betaine is a real lifesaver for many homocystinurics because when it's absent other interventions may not be effective. In any case, nutritional intervention with methylating supplements brings about dramatic improvement in homocystinuria—so much so that many patients can live largely normal lives.

Betaine packaged specifically for the high-dose treatment of homocystinurics is classified as a drug. It's called Cystadane.

Older people who have homocystinuria often receive specific benefits when treated with methyl-boosting supplementation. These include improvements in skin texture and hair pigmentation (vitamin B_6 therapy can darken and soften the coarse blond hair that's often a feature of homocystinuria) and, perhaps more important, the lowering of blood pressure and reduction or even elimination of the risk of excessive, life-threatening, blood clotting. Methyl supplementation will also relieve a whole array of psychiatric and nervous system disorders.

Although homocystinuria is a rare disorder, it offers clues as to the possible outcomes of lifelong moderately elevated levels of HCY. For example, moderately elevated HCY—say, 15 to 100 micromolar—is a risk for vascular disease, thrombosis, and depression, as well as a number of neurological and psychiatric disorders. Moderately elevated HCY has been suggested as a possible contributor to osteoporosis, and deficient methylation appears to contribute to cataracts. The elderly are often afflicted with one or all of these same disorders, implying that the same nutritional intervention used to treat homocystinuria is useful in smaller doses to lower HCY in "normal" people. In other words, *Methyl Magic* in large doses can treat extreme deficiencies in methylation that cause homocystinuria, but in smaller doses it can lower the less extreme levels of HCY and thus help prevent and even treat the ailments that can arise when HCY is moderately high.

Homocystinuria is an extreme example of what can happen when methylation goes awry. Methylation, as we've seen, is one of the cornerstones of life itself. If methylation is normal, life chugs along and the great dance of evolution goes on. But when methylation is deficient, the results can be anywhere from simply annoying to downright disastrous. In the ensuing chapters we'll take a hard, detailed look at what happens when methylation goes wrong.

CHAPTER 10

HEART DISEASE AND STROKE

Heart disease is tragic enough when it strikes people in old age, but in the rare instances when heart troubles victimize children, the event is not just tragic—it's absolutely bizarre. As such, childhood heart disease—especially arteriosclerosis—is in itself a living laboratory, a crucible in which scientists can observe key factors that may be triggering the malady, not only in children, but in people of all ages.

One scientist who has devoted much of his career to studying heart disease in children is Kilmer McCully, M.D. Now a pathologist at the Veterans Affairs Medical Center in Providence, Rhode Island, he was working at Harvard Medical School in the late 1960s when his story (and to some degree ours) began. At the time, McCully was studying specific cases of infants and children with rare genetic diseases called *inborn errors of metabolism*. These diseases left their victims unable to use certain vitamins in the same way normal children do. Results: mental retardation, eye lens dislocation, osteoporosis, and a variety of other problems. But perhaps the most striking effect was severe and almost inevitably fatal arteriosclerosis.

McCully examined a few of these afflicted children. Even with these few, because he understood the metabolism and pathology, McCully had a vital realization, one that still echoes today and is slowly changing the way we look at heart disease. McCully noticed that all of these cases of arteriosclerosis that resulted from inborn errors of metabolism had one factor in common. Each was marked by very high levels of HCY. Compared with normal people, these children had HCY levels that were vastly higher. In other words, these children all had homocystinuria. To McCully, the conclusion was inescapable: Very high levels of HCY, such as those found in these genetically diseased children, were the cause of vascular disease, stroke, and heart disease. He went on to reason that even moderately high levels of HCY, as in hyperhomocysteinemia—a condition that affects many of us but remains hidden unless we're tested for it specifically— may bring on heart disease and stroke in a more gradual way as we grow older.

It would be more than thirty years before the work of McCully and others on the role of HCY in heart disease began to make headlines. In the meantime, most research focused on the role of cholesterol. That focus kept the eyes of the scientific and medical communities—to say nothing of the media, government agencies, and public consciousness—squarely on cholesterol as the head villain in the heart disease story.

But little by little scientists began to follow up McCully's pioneering work by looking more closely at the relationship between high levels of HCY and heart disease. Prospective studies, in which blood is collected and people are charted for several years, show that elevated HCY was present in many people *before* they ever had a heart attack or stroke. Still other experiments showed that HCY stimulated the growth of *vascular smooth muscle cells (VSMC)*. Excessive growth of VSMC is one of the most basic events in arteriosclerosis.

Arteriosclerosis (and its cousin, atherosclerosis) is, of course, one of the major contributors to heart disease and stroke. One of the most fundamental events in arteriosclerosis is proliferation of VSMC into the connective tissue near the inside of blood vessels. This causes expansion of this tissue, narrowing of the inside of the blood vessel, and thus reduced blood flow. Another common event in arteriosclerosis is loss of the endothelial cells that line the inside of the blood vessel. These cells help avoid clotting and invasion of other cell types from the blood into the wall of the blood vessel.

The following figure is a cutaway diagram of an artery. The artery on the left is normal. In the middle artery, vascular smooth muscle cells have begun to invade the thin layer of connective tissue near the inside of the artery wall—an early step in the blocking of the artery that defines arteriosclerosis. In the diagram on the right the artery is in an advanced stage of arteriosclerosis, almost entirely blocked.

To study the possible role of HCY in arteriosclerosis at the cellular level, one team of researchers grew VSMC and endothelial cells with HCY at concentrations similar to those in blood plasma with hyperhomocysteinemia or homocystinuria. The results of their experiments showed that growth promotion of VSMC by HCY, and growth inhibition of endothelial cells, is one mechanism by which HCY could cause arteriosclerosis in humans and animals. Thus these researchers showed that at the cellular level HCY could indeed be a cause of vascular disease that can lead to heart attack and stroke.

One of the most useful ways to measure the progression of vascular disease—because it can highlight risk of a life-threatening stroke or heart attack before it's too late—is to study *stenosis*. Stenosis is narrowing of the inside of the arteries due to the thickening of the arterial wall caused by the growth of vascular smooth muscle cells, the deposit of fat in the arterial wall, or the calcification of the arterial wall. Stenosis can and does happen throughout the arterial system, but most often doctors are concerned with stenosis in specific arteries—the aorta, which leads directly from the heart to the body, and in the carotid arteries in the neck,

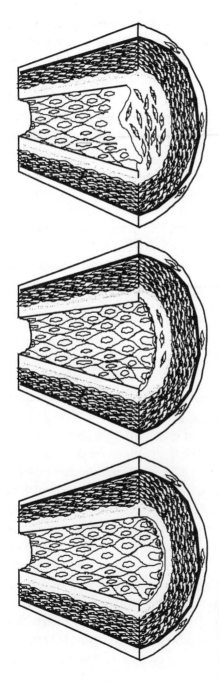

Arteriosclerosis

This figure shows a cutaway diagram of an artery: normal (*left*); beginning arteriosclerosis (*middle*); and advanced, leading to occlusion (*right*). In arteriosclerosis vascular smooth muscle cells invade the thin layer of connective tissue just near the inside of the vessel wall and expand it. The result is progressive thickening and distortion of the inside wall of this artery. Thickening and distortion of the artery interior can also involve fatty deposits (atherosclerosis) and calcification. Thickening and distortion make the artery inflexible so that it can't expand enough as blood is pumped through it. Thickening and distortion also makes an artery very narrow inside, constricting the flow of blood and inviting artery blockage.

which carry vital blood supplies to the brain. Stenosis can be a killer. If it takes place in the coronary arteries supplying the heart, it can ultimately lead to a fatal heart attack. If it takes place in the carotid arteries, the result can be a crippling or killer stroke.

If that weren't bad enough, stenosis limits blood circulation and increases the likelihood that a clot will block a blood vessel. Again, the potential result is heart attack or stroke. Stenosis probably causes HCY to accumulate in peripheral tissues and make arteriosclerosis even worse. Stenosis also causes high blood pressure because it reduces the flexibilty, and the elasticity, of your blood vessels. This in turn can lead to congestive heart failure and stroke, both potential killers. Even if stenosis doesn't kill you outright, it will slow down your circulation, and this in itself can have ugly consequences. Poor circulation can cause periodic lameness and can limit how much you can exert yourself.

Stenosis can take place in many of the body's arteries, but when it occurs in the carotid arteries physicians and scientists can study it more readily. That's because unlike most other arteries, the carotid arteries in the neck can be measured noninvasively for thickening, using ultrasound. This noninvasive measure, as well as the importance of the carotid arteries in supplying blood to the brain, make the carotids good arteries to study for the effects of HCY. During the 1990s a number of reseachers studied carotid artery wall thickening in relation to HCY. The earliest of these studies showed that high levels of HCY were indeed associated with carotid artery atherosclerosis and that this thickening of the carotid arteries occurred in patients who had not yet shown any outward symptoms of impending heart diease or stroke.

These initial studies were done with small numbers of patients. Then Jacob Selhub, Ph.D., at the USDA Human Nutrition Research Center on Aging (HNRCA) at Tufts University in Boston, and his co-workers examined more than one thousand people over the age of sixty-six for the degree of thickening of their carotid arteries. These people were then divided into two groups: those with the greatest thickening of their carotid arteries and those with the least. *People with high HCY levels were over twice as likely to be in the group with the greatest amount of thickening of the carotid arteries.* The group with the less thickened carotid arteries had on average lower levels of HCY. Interestingly enough, they also had the highest blood levels of methylating nutrients such as folate and the HCY-lowering nutrient vitamin B_6.

Animal studies of HCY have been equally revealing. In these experiments scientists have fed lab animals (rats, rabbits, and baboons) either methyl-deficient diets or diets high in either HCY or methionine. (In some cases researchers have taken a more direct route, by giving animals injections of HCY or methionine.) The results helped confirm what had been discovered in humans—arteriosclerosis, atherosclerosis, calcification, and dangerously excessive blood clotting. In many cases these animals died prematurely, either from these conditions or from related complications. Even more startling, these studies also show that methyl-deficient/methionine-excessive diets were *more likely to produce vascular disease than high-fat diets.*

All this evidence points strongly to a direct link between high levels of HCY and heart or vascular disease. The case for this link has been strengthened by other, more indirect evidence. For example, it's now known that there are many parallels between HCY and vascular disease. Both increase with age, while both are associated with males in general and with women during and after menopause. There are also several disease states where elevated HCY is also correlated with vascular disease. In the type of mental retardation known as Down's syndrome, for instance, in which HCY is very *low,* there is much less vascular disease.

HCY was eventually implicated in another basic aspect of vascular disease. Besides arteriosclerosis, HCY may play a role in an increased propensity for blood to clot and to form loose clots (known as *thrombi*) that circulate through the blood vessels. When a thrombus meets an area in an artery that is narrowed by arteriosclerosis, this can lead to blockage of the artery. Also the thickened tissue that narrows arteries can rupture and lead to clotting and blockage. Often this artery blockage leads directly to a fatal heart attack or stroke.

Even though high HCY is correlated with vascular disease, the relationship is not entirely clear-cut. Some people with moderately high HCY don't have vascular disease, while others who do have vascular disease don't have high HCY. Future, more definitive testing may help explain this anomaly by looking at levels of SAM, methylfolate, and other ingredients of methyl metabolism. It may turn out that either high HCY *or* low SAM is a risk factor for, or cause of, vascular disease.

It is also possible that HCY has what scientists call a *graded effect*. That is, HCY may be a risk factor for vascular disease even when HCY is low (say, 6 or 8 micromolar). Obviously, higher HCY (for example, 16 or 20 micromolar) would represent a higher risk, but lower HCY would still represent some, although perhaps less, risk. On the other hand, HCY may have what's known as a *threshold effect*. This would mean that below a certain level (say, less than 10 micromolar), HCY doesn't cause or contribute to vascular disease.

I suggest that HCY has a graded effect and propose that even normal levels (such as 10 micromolar) cause vascular disease. This would be consistent with what we know about evolution, in that normal levels could be harmful provided that the accumulated damage doesn't catch up to us until well after we have reproduced and raised children. Still, the damage could be occurring silently all the while, without precipitating a fatal or disabling event until after the children are raised.

Here's the bottom line: By now hundreds of studies, including the famous Framingham Heart Study, the Physicians Health Study, the Hordaland Homocysteine Study, and many, many others, have shown that elevated HCY is a risk factor for heart disease and stroke. Some studies credit HCY with causing only 5 to 20 percent of vascular disease. However, if HCY, or something closely related, such as low SAM, is an actual cause of vascular disease, then HCY may in fact cause as much as 90 percent of vascular disease. If that's so—and as we've said, many studies point in that direction—then *HCY is as great a risk factor for these diseases as is cholesterol, perhaps greater. In fact, high HCY is now widely recognized by scientists to be the greatest single biochemical risk factor for heart disease.*

Despite the evidence gathered in these studies, scientists still debate whether or not moderately elevated levels of HCY have been proven to cause vascular disease. Some scientists think HCY actually causes vascular disease; many don't think there's enough evidence yet. Nevertheless, many scientists and physicians now take folic acid and other supplements just to be on the safe side. None of this is to say that cholesterol and other factors play no role in the onset of heart disease. Certainly people with inborn errors of metabolism causing very high cholesterol also have vascular disease. It's seldom that a single factor is responsible for disease or health—especially when we're talking about age-related infirmities like heart disease and stroke. Usually a combination of factors—some nutritional, some genetic, some environmental, others having to do with overall lifestyle—is important. This is obviously true of heart disease and stroke. Cholesterol, fat, protein, and folic acid play important roles in setting the stage for these diseases, as do a number of other factors.

Still, the circumstantial evidence for a direct link between high HCY levels and heart disease, vascular disease, and stroke keeps mounting. Ongoing studies looking at the effects of folic acid supplements on second stroke, as well as a number of other studies in which methylating supplements are used to lower HCY, should help give us a definitive answer to this all-important question.

RELATED DISEASES

The havoc wreaked by high HCY levels and the resulting vascular disease isn't necessarily limited to heart disease and stroke. High HCY may play a part in the development of other diseases as well. Diabetes and kidney failure are two examples. Victims of both these ailments often have increased vascular disease and higher than normal levels of HCY. So far the evidence is sparse for a direct or causal connection between HCY and diabetes or renal failure, but many experts think that HCY contributes to the increased occurrence of vascular disease that accompanies these diseases.

DETERMINING HCY LEVELS

What determines our HCY levels? Two key players: genetics and nutrition. Some unfortunate people are genetically "built" to have inefficient versions of one or more of the enzymes that metabolize HCY and thus keep the levels in the safe range. Even if this genetic predisposition doesn't bring on full-blown homocystinuria, it can result in higher than normal levels of HCY, the condition known as hyperhomocysteinemia. As we've said, these unsafe levels of HCY are certainly a risk factor and probably a cause of heart disease, stroke, thrombosis, and other potentially fatal or disabling vascular diseases.

At present, tests for these unlucky genetic predispositions do exist, but they're highly specialized. Usually doctors or scientists perform these tests only on children or young adults who have very premature vascular disease. In the future, though—especially given the burgeoning awareness of HCY's role in heart disease—such tests could and should become far more routine. When that happens, the genetic risk factor for high HCY can be caught early, in childhood, well before vascular disease becomes life-threatening. The patient will then be able to take preventive measures, including a *Methyl Magic* regimen, to help halt the advance of heart disease.

People with nutritional deficiencies can be just as vulnerable to high HCY levels and its hazards as those with unfortunate genetic makeups. If intake of folate, vitamin B_6, vitamin B_{12}, and other methylating nutrients is low, then risk of high HCY and heart disease, stroke, thrombosis, or other vascular disease may also be high. Numerous studies with animals show that methyl-deficient diets or injections of HCY or methionine cause arteriosclerosis, which, as we've said so often, is often a prelude to heart disease. Those who have a combination of a genetic predisposition to high HCY and poor nutrition—especially poor methyl nutrition—obviously run a double hazard.

But even in this worst-case scenario, a change to healthier nutritional habits will nearly always lower HCY, thus reducing the risk of heart disease, stroke, thrombosis, or other vascular disease. The fortunate truth is that HCY levels are easy to control. For many people, simply taking a well-balanced multivitamin will do the trick. For many others, a focus on the methylating supplements in *Methyl Magic* will do an exquisite job of keeping HCY levels in the safe range.

LOWERING HCY

How low can HCY levels go, and what are the optimal levels for preventing disease and promoting good health? While the answers to these important questions aren't yet crystal clear, we do have some information on how much HCY can be reduced. In one study of elderly people (aged seventy-two to eighty), HCY was reduced with vitamin-supplement injections from the 11-to-14-micromolar range to about 8 micromolar. (By the way, 8 micromolar is lower than levels found in normal, healthy thirty-five-year-olds.) At the other end of the age spectrum, a study of people in their early twenties showed that HCY reduced from about 9.6 micromolar to about 7.26 micromolar after six weeks of 1.0 milligram folic acid, 400 micrograms vitamin B_{12}, and 10 milligrams B_6 per day. In another group HCY went from about 8.4 micromolar to about 5.6 micromolar after the same treatment.

METHYL MAGIC AND HEART DISEASE

If sluggish methyl metabolism puts one at risk of developing heart disease and its related diseases such as peripheral vascular disease, stroke, and so on, can one lower that risk by taking *Methyl Magic* supplements? A growing number of scientists, myself among them, think the answer may well be a resounding yes.

Many researchers now recognize and promote vitamin supplements as an easy way to lower HCY. Their recommendations often include folic acid, vitamins B_6 and B_{12}, and betaine—among the very supplements I've highlighted in this book. In fact, a recent study at the Cleveland Clinic suggested that as much as one-fifth of the American population—that's more than fifty million people—may be at increased risk for heart attack and stroke because they're not getting enough folic acid and vitamin B_6. At the same time, scientists at the University of Maryland found that high doses of vitamins B_6 and B_{12} along with folic acid significantly lowered blood levels of HCY and also raised levels of a substance called *thrombomodulin*, part of the body's natural defense system against the formation of life-threatening blood clots.

But how much of these supplements should you take? What's the ideal amount to keep HCY in check and maintain your methyl metabolism at optimally healthy rates? Scientists have tested a wide range of doses. Folic acid studies, for example, have used amounts varying from 400 to 5,000 micrograms a day. Vitamin B_6 studies have looked at doses ranging from 5 to 50 milligrams, while those that focused on vitamin B_{12} have used amounts between 400 and 1,000 micrograms. Betaine studies have used grams a day. But you don't have to go to the extreme high end of these test doses to get the benefits of *Methyl Magic*. For most people the amounts recommended in chapter 5 will do very nicely. Stick to that regimen and you'll soon see results such as weight loss, more energy and stamina, and increased mental alertness. All these are signposts of profound changes taking place in your body. I'm convinced that changes such as lowered HCY, increased SAM, and a smoothly running methyl metabolism are the keys to preventing heart disease and its gang of killer relatives.

CHAPTER 11

CANCER

I f methylation and methyl metabolism play a central role in heart disease—still the number one killer in America—is it also implicated in our number two killer, cancer? The answer may well be "yes." A growing body of research, particularly in the last decade, indicates that low methylation rates may be cancer's handmaiden and perhaps one of its causes.

DNA METHYLATION AND CANCER

As early as 1977 a Russian team looked at normal cells from cows, then compared those with cells from cows who had a type of cancer known as *lympholeukemia*. In general, the overall DNA methylation was lower in cells from the animals with cancer. This was one of the early clues that methylation—DNA methylation, at least—might be involved in cancer, either as a cause or as a result.

However, would the same findings hold up in *Homo sapiens*? Over the next twenty years a number of studies in humans have shown that overall, DNA methylation decreases as cancers develop. One group of studies involving nearly one hundred patients showed that normal tissues had the highest DNA methylation levels. As tissues began to move in the direction of the uncontrolled growth that defines cancer, DNA methylation decreased at each stage. In other words, methylation levels were lower in benign tumors than in normal tissues. They were lower still in cancerous tumors and lowest of all in cancers that had already spread to other parts of the body (metastatic cancer).

Another important clue came with the discovery that rats with low methylation rates have an abnormally large amount of breakage in their DNA strands. Some of that breakage occurs in a gene known as *p53*, which normally helps suppress the growth of cancerous tumors.

Declining DNA methylation has been studied in most detail in colon cancer. Here again, scientists have discovered that the progression of cancer development from normal tissue to benign tumor to malignant tumor is marked by progressive loss of DNA methylation. Yet there's an apparent paradox here. In some cancer cells specific DNA sequences become *more* methylated as cancers develop. These seemingly contradictory processes may take place because the cells' overall regulation of DNA methylation is thrown out of whack as cancers develop. Still, in these cases the overall DNA methylation levels nearly always drop.

NUTRITION, METHYLATION, AND CANCER IN THE LABORATORY

If you've read this far, you already know that the food we eat—and especially the supplements we take—have a great deal to do with our bodies' ability to carry on normal methylation, whether it's methyl metabolism in general or DNA methylation in particular. Does the same apply to cancer? Can poor methyl nutrition bring on cancer? Can cancer be treated by the *Methyl Magic* program?

Here again, there's considerable evidence that the answers to these questions may be a hopeful "yes." More than fifty years ago scientists began experimenting with feeding animals methyl-deficient diets. A great many of these experiments showed that nutritional deficiency in choline and methionine—two key players in methyl metabolism—cause cancer in a number of animal species. Often these experimental animals have methyl-deficient diets marked by low concentrations not only of choline and methionine, but also of folic acid and/or vitamin B_{12}.

In 1946 scientists found that rats fed a diet low in methionine and free of choline had more liver cancer than rats eating a normal diet. Unfortunately these researchers used an extracted peanut meal as part of the low-methionine, no-choline diet. As a result, other scientists quibbled for years, arguing that a toxin from a peanut fungus may have been the real cause of the cancer. But the controversy was resolved eventually when more and more experiments showed that indeed dietary methyl deficiency caused cancer in rats and in mice. Dietary methyl deficiency can also be mimicked by feeding animals *ethionine*, a substance that inhibits methyl metabolism.

Why does methyl deficiency cause cancer in these animals? Methyl-deficient diets reduce concentrations of SAM in the liver. They also raise concentrations of S-adenosylhomocysteine (SAH), a component of methyl metabolism that, if elevated, inhibits methylation reactions and can also lead to elevated levels of HCY. These low SAM levels and high SAH levels generally limit methylation of DNA and other molecules. In the liver, for example, low methylation of DNA means that oncogenes—the genes that help start the cancer process in motion—lose methylation and are "switched on" at a higher than normal rate. If these oncogenes are "turned up" high enough in cells, it will drive cell growth and proliferation and will eventually lead to cancer. Methyl deficiency also results in fatty accumulation in the livers of animals—a warning sign for cancer.

PREVENTING CANCER WITH METHYL MAGIC

If methyl deficiency can cause cancer, it seems reasonable to think that correcting the deficiency might help prevent or even treat the disease. Indeed, a number of exciting studies suggest this possibility. Some of these studies show that supplementation of rats with SAM can increase DNA methylation in precancerous tissue and can maintain DNA methylation under conditions in which it might otherwise be lost.

For example, scientists can bring on cancer development in lab animals by injecting them with various cancer-causing substances. This first creates precancerous nodules in the liver, which are usually low in methylation and consequently high in oncogene expression. With oncogenes thus being "switched on" at an accelerated rate, these nodules can later develop into full-blown cancer tumors.

When precancerous nodules were thus initiated in rats, scientists then gave them supplements of SAM. The results were striking: The precancerous nodules returned to a more normal type of tissue, and the oncogenes in these liver nodule cells were "turned down." As a result, cell proliferation in these precancerous nodules slowed. Overall, DNA methylation in these liver nodule cells increased, especially in several potentially dangerous oncogenes. The ultimate payoff: These SAM-supplemented rats had a much lower incidence of liver cancer than rats not treated with SAM. Other studies have demonstrated that feeding betaine to rats also increases production of SAM in their livers. Dr. Anthony Barak and others have demonstrated that betaine fed to rats will increase their liver SAM and decrease fat accumulation in their livers. But it is not yet known whether betaine supplementation alone can prevent any kind of cancer.

METHYL METABOLISM, DNA METHYLATION, AND POSSIBLE CANCER PREVENTION IN HUMANS

When all is said and done, of course, rats are rats and humans are humans. There are many genetic similarities among mice, rats, and men; however, there are also many differences. So the only way to establish a method of prevention or treatment with any degree of certainty is to study humans. That's especially true of cancer, in which many treatments that have shown promise in rats have ultimately failed in humans.

In humans, the primary target of DNA methylation studies and nutritional treatments in this area has been colon cancer and the precancerous polyps that often precede full-blown cancer. It's been found that in general DNA methylation decreases as cancer develops. At the same time, DNA methylation *increases* on so-called tumor suppressor genes. So in many respects colon cancer development in humans does follow the same molecular pathway as does liver cancer development in methyl-deficient rats.

Two of the most revealing studies in humans, conducted by researchers at Harvard Medical School, have been the Nurses Health Study and the Health Professionals Follow-Up Study. These were important because they involved large numbers of people—over 15,000 women and more than 9,000 men—and because many individuals were examined *before* any cancer had been detected. Volunteers who were found to have precancerous polyps in their colons (564 women and 331 men) were then compared with the larger groups for a number of telltale factors. In the end, the Harvard team identified three new risk factors for precancerous polyps in the colon. One was high consumption of alcohol. The other two—low folate and low methionine—were directly related to methylation and indicated that in these patients methylation rates might be dangerously low. At the same time, those who had the *highest* folate and methionine and *lowest* alcohol consumption had much lower incidence of colon polyps (only 2.7 percent) compared with the average for the general population (an estimated 10 percent of men over forty years of age).

Still, interestingly enough, almost none of these subjects had folate so low as to be considered medically deficient. Medical folate deficiency is usually defined as blood levels less than 2.6 nanograms of folate per milliliter of blood plasma or serum. Remember, most of the volunteers in this study were health professionals and so probably less likely to be medically deficient in folate than subjects in the general population. But even among those who had "sufficient" levels of folate, there was a wide variation in the incidence of colon and rectal polyps. The researchers also noted that folate intake from foods only (excluding supplements) was at best only weakly associated with decreased risk of polyps in the colon and rectum.

In further work on the Nurses Health Study researchers have shown, this time with colon cancer, that folic acid intake of at least 400 micrograms per day reduced risk. In particular this research points to long-term use of multivitamin supplements containing folic acid for protection against colon cancer. Meanwhile a 1994 study has shown that folic acid supplements help maintain DNA methylation in the tissue (mucous membrane) that lines the rectum.

But there is more evidence for an association between folate levels and cancer, evidence that suggests folic acid may well help prevent other cancers in humans. Bruce Ames, Ph.D., and his colleagues at the University of California at Berkeley studied people who were folate deficient and those with normal folate levels. They tested these people for DNA damage, which can lead to cancer. Their studies showed that people with low folate in their blood had DNA damage at levels eight times that of people with normal folate levels. The Ames team then treated the deficient and normal folate individuals with 5 milligrams (5,000 micrograms) of folic acid per day for eight weeks. They showed that treatment with folic acid supplements increased blood folates in both the originally folate-deficient and originally normal individuals, so that after supplementation both groups had about the same blood folate levels. This increase in blood folates was accompanied by a *twentyfold decrease* in DNA damage in those people who had previously been folate deficient. Those who had normal folate levels before supplementation still showed a threefold decrease in DNA damage. This shows that folate supplementation can have important cancer-preventing effects—even in people with so-called normal folate levels.

Several subsequent studies have also shown that high folate, high B_{12} and low HCY levels help prevent DNA damage. Again even high versus low levels of folate within the "normal" range are important. Another recent study, reported in 1998, shows that folic acid also helps to maintain DNA methylation in white blood cells.

These results again raise the question of optimum levels of folic acid and other nutrients in the diet. While these have yet to be established scientifically, I think the recommendations for folic acid in the *Methyl Magic* program may help us reach the optimal levels that may in turn help prevent cancer.

Taken together, these groundbreaking studies give a generous boost to the case that folic acid is a key player in the prevention of cancer. Folate supplements are apparently the most effective way to raise folate intake enough to lower the risk of these cancers. In other words, using just one of the tricks in your *Methyl Magic* bag—taking daily supplements of folic acid—may spare you the agony of cancer.

It may well be that other aspects of your *Methyl Magic* program could be just as helpful as folic acid supplements in your battle to prevent cancer. Some other nutrients that need more study include choline and betaine. Fruits and vegetables clearly reduce the risk of colon cancer, and many of these contain significant amounts of choline. Some also contain significant amounts of betaine. But betaine and choline, even though they obviously have an important impact on methyl metabolism, have not been studied as cancer preventives as systematically as have folic acid and methionine.

TREATMENT OF CANCER

It's possible, perhaps even likely, that in the future the same methyl-boosting strategies that can help prevent cancer may also help treat the disease. Such treatment might combine extensive modification of the diet, judicious use of methylating supplements, and very specific chemotherapies designed to halt and destroy cancers. In theory all this is possible. If one could control the folate cycles that the body uses both to make methyl groups and to manufacture the "building blocks" for DNA, then control of cell growth should follow. Since cancer is essentially a disease in which cells grow seemingly without limit, putting the brakes to that uncontrolled growth should stop the disease itself. Indeed, this is what chemotherapy is designed to do. But with a few notable exceptions, chemotherapy alone has at best a mediocre record in beating back cancer.

Still, we don't yet know how to devise a *Methyl Magic* program that will undo cancer once it's started. The recommendations in this book for normal, healthy people—or even for people with a variety of health problems—are not necessarily good for those with cancer. There's always the danger that this sort of intervention may give already developed cancers an extra growth spurt. So before we use *Methyl Magic* to treat (as opposed to preventing) human cancer, we really need much more research in which methylating strategies and chemotherapies are used to treat animals. For example, folic acid has been used to improve the effectiveness and reduce the side effects of chemotherapy in rats. These approaches hold great potential and should be pursued and worked out in the laboratory.

One such approach involves the use of choline. This nutrient may be important in treating cancer not only because it's a methyl donor, but because it's a key component in the "cellular switchboard" that regulates the chemical signaling system in the membranes of our cells. Regulation of this intracellular communication system has long been recognized as important in cancer development. Some experts think that choline deficiency can cause glitches in this communication system and that these glitches may contribute to the onset of cancer.

Until more research is done, the question as to whether or not *Methyl Magic* will become an ingredient in cancer treatment remains unanswered. But the theory is in place, and some of the early experimental signs seem positive. In the meantime, it seems apparent that *Methyl Magic* can be a powerful weapon in preventing cancer.

CHAPTER 12

ARTHRITIS AND LUPUS

We've seen that low methylation rates almost certainly play a part in the development of heart disease and cancer. Low methylation may also cause three other diseases: rheumatoid arthritis, osteoarthritis, and lupus. Among them, these debilitating ailments afflict more than eighteen million Americans.

Rheumatoid arthritis and lupus are marked in particular by loss of DNA methylation. In fact, other than cancer and aging (we'll tackle the latter in chapter 15), rheumatoid arthritis and lupus are the only diseases in which a loss of DNA methylation is clearly part and parcel of the ailments. Heart disease and other ailments discussed in this book are associated with low methylation rates in general, but not necessarily with low methylation of DNA. As with cancer and aging, the case for low DNA methylation is supported by a large number of test tube experiments with animal cells.

RHEUMATOID ARTHRITIS

Rheumatoid arthritis (RA) is characterized by stiff joints, especially in the morning, as well as by swelling, inflamation, and tenderness in the joints. The actual cause of RA is unknown, but it appears to be at least in part a disease in which the immune system turns traitor and begins to attack the body's own tissues—in this case the tissues in the joints.

(Diseases in which the immune system turns against the body are known as *autoimmune diseases.*)

The connection between RA and low methylation rates—especially low rates of DNA methylation—has been the subject of intense scientific scrutiny. For example, Dr. Bruce Richardson and colleagues at the University of Michigan, Ann Arbor, have shown that patients with RA have lower white blood cell (specifically T-cell) DNA methylation than do healthy people. Another study yielded similar results, but with the added kicker that patients whose RA was in remission actually had higher DNA methylation than people who had never had the disease. (Soon afterward yet another study revealed that RA patients who were treated with methotrexate—a drug that suppresses the immune system and inhibits cell growth—also had higher rates of DNA methylation than normal, healthy people.)

With the case for the connection between RA and low DNA methylation rates growing ever stronger, scientists began to look for links between RA and other telltale signs of low methylation rates in general. One study at the USDA Human Nutrition Research Center on Aging (HNRCA) at Tufts University in Boston examined levels of folate, vitamin B_{12}, and vitamin B_6 in these patients and found only B_6 to be lower in RA patients than in people who didn't have the disease. The HNRCA team then looked at HCY levels, comparing twenty-eight RA patients with twenty healthy volunteers. The researchers measured fasting HCY levels as well as HCY after a standard methionine load (methionine-loading test). In both tests HCY was higher in RA patients than in healthy volunteers. Seeing the results, the researchers suggested that a combination of methylating supplements—folate, vitamin B_6, and vitamin B_{12}—might be helpful in treating RA.

OSTEOARTHRITIS

Osteoarthritis (OA) is a degeneration and loss of cartilage in the joints. Cartilage acts as a sort of biological "shock absorber" and keeps the bones in the joints from rubbing against one another. If that cartilage is lost or damaged, the result can be fatigue fractures in the underlying bone. These fractures lead to repair, which in turn brings increased growth of the bone. That makes the disease worse. It's estimated that tens of millions of Americans have evidence of OA; this includes a large majority of people over seventy. Even in people over fifty, OA is responsible for a great deal of pain and disability.

Let's turn the microscope up a bit so that we can take a deeper look at what happens to bring on OA. In OA there is a reduction in the size of molecules called *proteoglycans*, which are the fundamental building blocks that make up cartilage. These proteoglycans are found in component cartilage cells known as *chondrocytes*. Experts think that as proteoglycans shrink, cartilage in the joints loses some of its ability to compress. (It's as if the shock absorbers in your car stiffened, giving you a bumpier ride.) To compensate, the body produces more chondrocytes and more cartilage. But the body can't quite keep up with the loss of cartilage owing to the shrinking of proteoglycans. The result is more cartilage loss and more severe OA.

An important clue to the role of methylation in OA turned up in studies conducted during the middle to late 1970s, when scientists began to look at SAM as a possible weapon in the battle against depression (see chapter 14). As is often the case in medical science, these studies turned up a surprise bonus. Some patients in these depression studies also had OA and it turns out that SAM, which was effective in treating depression, simultaneously relieved OA symptoms.

Following the trail, researchers, especially in Germany and Italy, mounted a number of trials to look specifically at SAM as a treatment for OA. Happily, it turned out that SAM reduced the symptoms of OA—in fact, it did so at least as effectively as ibuprofen and other *nonsteroidal anti-inflammatory drugs (NSAIDs)*, including good old aspirin. (This is because SAM increases production of proteoglycans at the same time it increases methylation.) Tens of thousands of patients have been involved in these studies, and trials as long as two years showed that SAM remained effective against OA.

Other research has focused on replacing those limited proteoglycans with a dietary supplement known as *glucosamine sulfate*. Although not a methyl supplement, glucosamine may be a component that helps facilitate proteoglycan repair. Thus glucosamine sulfate may be necessary for effective treatment of OA. More studies are certainly needed, but it appears that the most effective relief of OA is likely to come from a combination treatment using either SAM or *Methyl Magic* supplements along with glucosamine sulfate.

The *Methyl Magic* program may confer the added benefit of helping OA patients control their weight. If you're carrying extra weight, you're putting an extra load on joints that are already worn. A number of studies indicate that weighing less will help minimize OA, especially in weight-bearing joints such as the knees. Keep in mind that NSAIDs like aspirin and ibuprofen, which are commonly used to treat OA, will relieve pain and inflammation but don't provide the material to rebuild or repair damaged tissues in the joints.

LUPUS

Lupus refers to a group of autoimmune diseases in which your immune system attacks your own body, subjecting it to what might be called "friendly fire." Among the targets of this friendly fire are DNA and proteins on chromosomes, substances fundamental to life. Lupus is characterized by joint pain, muscle pain, central nervous system disorders, and a variety of other symptoms, including rash, fever, arthritis, and hair loss. Although in most cases the underlying cause of lupus is unknown, the disease can be brought on by drugs—including procainamide and quinidine, which are used to control certain kinds of heart arrhythmias, as well as hydralazine, which is prescribed for high blood pressure and congestive heart failure.

Like arthritis, lupus is linked to low methylation rates, especially methylation of DNA. A telltale clue: Some of the drugs that can bring on lupus also lower DNA methylation. A number of studies of patients with various types of lupus indicate that DNA methylation is low in certain immune system cells known as *monocytes*. Although the cause of lupus remains unknown, this and other evidence from animal experiments lead some experts to suspect that loss of DNA methylation is at least one of the causes of the disease.

To get a better handle on the link between methylation and diseases such as arthritis and lupus, researchers could monitor DNA methylation of blood cells in affected patients taking folic acid, B_{12}, SAM, or other methyl-boosting supplements. That way scientists could determine if these nutrients affect white blood cell DNA methylation and if such supplements improved patients' conditions. Such experiments might also help answer the question of whether or not low DNA methylation is a cause of RA or lupus. At the moment it's not known with certainty if methyl supplements will prevent or treat lupus or RA. Studies linking low folate with loss of DNA methylation in white blood cells (of which monocytes are one type) are encouraging and indicate that a good diet combined with supplements may well help prevent or reduce the severity of lupus. The fact that SAM seems to be of help in relieving symptoms of OA suggests that *Methyl Magic* supplements—designed to boost the body's production of SAM—may be of help to OA patients. Hopefully this will turn out to be true for RA as well.

CHAPTER 13

OTHER DISEASES

NERVOUS SYSTEM DISORDERS

I f you or someone you know is afflicted with fibromyalgia, chronic fatigue syndrome, or even multiple sclerosis—diseases that attack some component of the nervous system—you know, perhaps painfully well, how frightening and debilitating they can be. In that case, you may be intrigued to know that these diseases behave in some important ways like homocystinuria or other severe nutritional deficiencies of methyl-boosting nutrients: folate, vitamin B_{12}, and some others on the *Methyl Magic* list. In other words, it's highly likely that methyl deficiency plays a significant role in some or all of these disorders.

If that's so, there's good cause for hope that at least some cases of these diseases can be treated successfully with methyl-boosting strategies. SAM in particular has produced eye-opening results in treating some of these diseases of the nervous system.

FIBROMYALGIA

As much as 2 percent of all Americans suffer from *fibromyalgia*. That sounds small, but this is a big country, so were talking about some four *million* people. Fibromyalgia is more common in women than in men. It generally strikes in middle age, but the occurrences of it increase as we grow older. The telltale symptoms of fibromyalgia are widespread, chronic aching and stiffness in the muscles and bone, with various places on the body being painfully sensitive to pressure. If that weren't enough, there's a litany of other common and disruptive symptoms of the disease, including severe fatigue, sleep disturbance, headaches, abnormal sensations such as burning or itching, "allergic" symptoms, irritable bowel syndrome, and depression. In one study the majority of women with fibromyalgia experienced pain and fatigue during more than 90 percent of their waking hours.

No one has yet pinpointed the cause of fibromyalgia, though scientists have a number of ideas. It's possible, for example, that the disease is caused, or at least triggered, either by autoimmunity or viral infections.

Luckily doctors can treat some symptoms of fibromyalgia—including pain and sleep disturbance—and also improve the patient's general state of well-being with drugs. Antidepressants like Prozac or Elavil, or combinations of these and/or other antidepressants, can bring much needed relief. But these drugs can have unwanted side effects: sexual dysfunction in the case of Prozac; bowel disorders, anxiety, even high blood pressure and heart attack, among many others, in the case of Elavil.

But there may be a better way to treat fibromyalgia, using elements of *Methyl Magic*. A number of studies over the years have shown some hopeful results using SAM, vitamin B_{12}, or choline. In one of these studies researchers looked at eleven patients who met the criteria for both fibromyalgia and chronic fatigue syndrome. These patients all had quite elevated levels of HCY in their cerebrospinal fluid, almost five times normal levels, an intriguing tip-off that low methylation rates are a hallmark of these ailments. We should note, though, that more common measures such as blood plasma HCY and levels of folate and vitamin B_{12} were normal in most of these same patients. These abnormally high levels of HCY in cerebrospinal fluid were also correlated with ratings of exhaustion in these patients.

In an even more dramatic study, Italian researchers used SAM to treat seventeen patients with primary fibromyalgia. (Eleven of these patients were also significantly depressed.) SAM treatment produced a significant improvement not only in reducing the number of painful sites on the patients' bodies, but in relieving their depression as well. There were no such happy results with placebos. The Italian team concluded that in these patients there was a correspondence between the main physical and psychological disturbances in fibromyalgia and that SAM was an effective treatment for both.

These studies, of course, were conducted only on small numbers of patients. To my knowledge no one has systematically addressed the question of whether a consistent, broadly based, supplementation program—with an emphasis on methyl-boosting supplements—would normalize the HCY or raise SAM in fibromyalgia, or whether such a program would help large numbers of these patients. But the clues are certainly there. It's my guess that once large-scale studies are done, *Methyl Magic*, or at least some of its components, may well become an important feature in the treatment of this nasty disease.

CHRONIC FATIGUE SYNDROME

Millions of Americans complain that they're tired and listless much of the time. Some of these unfortunate people have *chronic fatigue syndrome* (*CFS*), a complex disease with a long list of symptoms. Not only are these patients so tired so often that they can't perform their daily activities, they may also suffer from muscle and joint pain, headache, mental confusion, depression, anxiety, and irritability.

Like fibromyalgia, the actual causes of CFS remain unknown. Some scientists think that the underlying cause may be a temporary weakness of the immune system. If exacerbated by emotional or physical stress, this weakness may allow viruses that have remained dormant in the body to "come to life," creating the disease and producing the symptoms.

One possible culprit is the Epstein-Barr virus. It's been found in some, but not all, patients suffering from CFS. Alternatively, some scientists propose that CFS is the result of imbalances in the immune system that crop up when it struggles against stress or allergies. The medical community is still experimenting with treatments for CFS. The major focus has been on drugs that enhance the immune system. But even these treatments have had limited success at best. A great many victims of CFS continue to struggle with the disease.

Like fibromyalgia, though, there are tantalizing hints that low methylation may play an important role in CFS. One study of sixty CFS patients revealed that at least half were clearly deficient in folic acid (blood plasma or blood serum levels below 3.0 micrograms per liter), while another 13 percent were borderline. In contrast, the scientists estimated that only 5 to 11 percent of the general population would have folate levels below 3.0 micrograms per liter. This team had previously shown that folate levels were low in patients suffering from influenza, mononucleosis, and mycoplasmal pneumonia—all infections caused by viruses or mycoplasmas. So in essence these studies helped establish a connection between poor methylation and infectious disease, and particularly with CFS.

Can *Methyl Magic* help treat CFS? The jury is still out. There have been few published studies, and results have sometimes been equivocal. To be fair, though, in some of these efforts patients were given, say, B_{12} without folic acid (or vice versa), so that the full effects of methylating supplementation were blunted, with consequently disappointing results. But since CFS is considered a subset of fibromyalgia, which can be treated with SAM, it's not unreasonable to think that *Methyl*

Magic supplementation might help alleviate CFS. So if you've been diagnosed with CFS, have your doctor check your HCY levels. If HCY is high or if folate and vitamin B_{12} levels are in the lower half of the normal range, you and your doctor might consider giving the *Methyl Magic* program a try.

MULTIPLE SCLEROSIS

Multiple sclerosis (MS) is a chronic, inflammatory, autoimmune disease in which the patient's immune system attacks proteins in the myelin sheath, which insulates the nerves and helps speed the conduction of electrical impulses that our nerves transmit. New research indicates that the disease also attacks the nerve fibers themselves. The symptoms of MS include weakness, fatigue, sensory loss, abnormal sensations, optic neuritis, double vision, vertigo, and a number of other neurological abnormalities. MS usually strikes people in their twenties to forties and is more likely to occur in women than in men.

In MS, patients undergo repeated attacks during which myelin is degraded. These attacks are often followed by periods of recovery as damaged myelin is repaired. Unfortunately the cycles of repair generally don't keep up with damage from the previous attacks. Pregnancy reduces the frequency of relapses in MS, but there is often an increase in the frequency of relapse in the mother after the baby is born. The progression of MS can be severe and sometimes fatal.

But hidden in this gruesome litany of symptoms are clues that MS may be linked to methylation. In particular, repair of the myelin sheath requires methylation as well as healthy oils. Also, as we've seen, poor methylation is associated with some other autoimmune diseases. Thus adequate methylation may be important both in the prevention of attacks as well as repair of damaged myelin.

This bears explanation. Myelin consists primarily of lipids (fats) and protein, including myelin basic protein. To do its job, myelin basic protein *must be methylated.* For the body to methylate, produce, or repair myelin, a number of essential nutrients are needed. Which nutrients? First, those that make up some of the lipids in the myelin sheath: monounsaturated, saturated, and essential fatty acids, such as those found in vegetables and in fat from cold-water fish. Second (although not necessarily in this order), the nutrients that aid in methylation, in this case methylation of myelin basic protein, and methylation to make phosphatidyl choline, also an essential component of membranes. That means folic acid, choline, and the rest of the *Methyl Magic* list.

MS is a frustratingly complex disease with a number of interwoven causes. *Magnetic resonance imaging (MRI)* can detect telltale MS lesions in the white matter within the brain and in the spinal cord. Inflammation and autoantibodies to myelin components are an important feature of MS attacks. Viral infection may also have a role, either as an initiating event or as an ongoing contributor.

It may be that nutritional deficits prevent myelin from ever being adequately repaired. It is also possible that inadequate nutrition has a role in the autoimmune aspects of MS. Many patients with MS have been shown to be deficient in vitamin B_{12} or folic acid. Other victims may have normal levels of vitamin B_{12} in their blood serum but low levels in the cerebrospinal fluid that bathes the brain and spinal cord. In fact, at least one study of a small number of MS patients has shown that those with the lowest serum B_{12} levels had the highest rate of disease progression. These patients also had low levels of folate. The researchers who conducted this study concluded that the vitamin B deficiency was either a result of treatment with steroids or was one of the causes of the disease itself. In some cases nutrient therapy does seem to help patients with MS.

Another clue to the role of poor methyl nutrition in MS comes from findings that patients with low levels of vitamin B_{12} in their blood or cerebrospinal fluid also had high levels of HCY. But in many cases patients have normal levels of HCY in their bloodstream. Only in the cerebrospinal fluid was HCY high. At the same time, these studies suggest that the cause of vitamin B_{12} deficiency in MS may be the body's inability to "latch on" to B_{12} and transport it to its proper destinations in the nervous system.

In any case, it seems important that MS patients should have both their blood plasma *and* cerebrospinal fluid tested for levels not only of HCY, but of other methylating substances like folate, vitamin B_{12}, and SAM. Likewise their white blood cell DNA methylation should be checked to determine if this may be a factor in the autoimmune component of MS, as it is with some other autoimmune diseases. Without this testing these potentially crucial aspects of the disease might be missed entirely.

While there is some evidence that MS may have a methyl-deficiency component, especially in the cerebrospinal fluid, there is even more evidence for a fat component. Particularly dangerous are diets high in saturated fat and low in unsaturated fats. More than fifty years ago a study showed that there were more cases of MS among inland Norwegians, who eat mainly saturated dairy fat, than among coastal Norwegians, who get most of their fats in monounsaturated or polyunsaturated form from eating mainly fish. Numerous subsequent studies support these findings. One expert, Roy Swank, M.D., Ph.D., of the Swank MS Treatment Clinic, Beaverton, Oregon, has for years advocated a low-fat diet supplemented with polyunsaturated fats as a treatment for MS. There are many reports of improvement in MS when his guidelines are followed.

So the weight of scientific evidence supports a connection between MS and shortages of nutrients, particularly methyl boosters like folate and vitamin B_{12}. It's apparent that without adequate nutritional support, damaged myelin can't be repaired, and this essential nutritional support will not necessarily be found in a "normal" diet. While we don't yet know the precise levels of methylating nutrients that will help stave off or treat MS, it makes sense to be sure that MS sufferers take in these nutrients in reasonable abundance. Actually, it may help these patients to maintain methyl-boosting nutrient levels, as well as mono- and polyunsaturated fats, on the high side of the normal range or higher. Keep in mind that the ravages of many other diseases can be reduced by maintaining higher than normal levels of certain vital nutrients.

Until we pinpoint the causes of some of these diseases, and determine the precise optimal levels of methylating nutrients that might help prevent or treat them, it only makes sense to be sure our bodies' own restorative efforts are supported by proper nutrition. This is especially important because some neurological disorders are easily mistaken for others, so that a specific treatment that works for one disease may not work for another or may even make it worse. If you have a nutritional defiency that is causing or exacerbating a disease, all the drugs in the world are not going to provide you with a definitive cure. It would be tragic if a patient who needed primarily nutrient therapy with methylating supplements like folic acid and vitamin B_{12} were instead treated only with drugs, perhaps leading to permanent neurological damage that might have been easily prevented.

ANEMIA

Most people associate anemia with low levels of iron. While iron deficiency can certainly be a cause of anemia, it should never be considered the sole cause without thorough testing. Treating low iron as the "cure-all" for anemia can have serious downsides. Most Western diets, especially those containing significant amounts of red meat—as in the United

States—probably err on the side of too much iron, especially for most adult men and postmenopausal women. In fact, people who take large doses of iron supplements over a long period of time run the risk of serious complications, including diarrhea, vomiting, diabetes, cirrhosis, and even heart failure. Still, all of us, especially young women and children, need adequate amounts of iron in our diet.

In any case, there can be a good deal more going on in anemia than simple iron deficiency. Once again, methylation levels and methylating nutrients may be important contributors both to the development of the disease and to its treatment. For example, low levels of folate or vitamin B_{12} have long been associated with anemia. In fact, severe forms of anemia are some of the first signs of B_{12} or folate deficiency. Iron supplements will not cure a folate or B_{12} deficiency.

If you have persistent fatigue or otherwise suspect that you're anemic, get a thorough medical exam. Be sure to ask your doctor to check your levels not only of iron, but also of HCY, vitamin B_{12}, and folate. If the levels of the latter two are low, even in the lower half of the normal range, your doctor may recommend that you take them as supplements. If your physician doesn't recommend these methylating supplements (some doctors are still in the dark concerning the role of HCY in disease, while others think we get all the vitamins we need from our food), then you may want to get a second, third, or even fourth opinion.

But if you do opt for a methyl-boosting approach, be sure you take both folate *and* vitamin B_{12}. There have been *very rare* instances in which patients with pernicious anemia due to B_{12} malabsorption and deficiency had progression of neurological symptoms when they were treated with folic acid alone, without vitamin B_{12}. In these cases, folic acid supplementation at high levels (generally much greater than 1 milligram per day) can mask pernicious anemia long enough to result in irreversible damage to the nervous system. That's just one reason we recommend that folic acid, B_{12}, and B_6 supplements all be taken as a group. If you like, you can even take them at the same time or in the same tablet.

ASTHMA AND ALLERGIC REACTIONS

Asthma, allergies, and several other conditions—including intestinal ailments like Crohn's disease and ulcerative colitis—all involve the release in the body of a substance known as *histamine*. In asthma, histamine release can choke and inflame the bronchial tubes, making it difficult to breathe. In allergy, a host of negative responses are triggered when organs in contact with the environment, such as the skin, respiratory tract, and gastrointestinal tract, come in contact with *allergens* (allergy-inducing substances), which in turn trigger the release of histamine and set the allergic response in motion.

The body regulates histamine through the action of two enzymes, the more important of which is called *histamine N-methyltransferase* (*HMT*). (High levels of HMT enzyme are found in the human kidney, intestine, brain, lung, and bronchial tubes.) It turns out that HMT uses SAM as a methyl donor. In other words, this enzyme is dependent on methyl metabolism for its ability to keep histamine in check.

The possibility that methyl deficiency could contribute to asthma and other allergic reactions should be investigated and could be very important. High levels of histamine release could create local methyl deficiency, which in turn could impair histamine metabolism and lead to a stronger allergic reaction. Increased levels of histamine or chronic histamine release would presumably require more methylation and lead to greater methyl deficiency. Thus a vicious circle might develop in which methylation never catches up to histamine release. In such a case a good way to promote recovery may be to make sure methylation is adequate by taking methyl-boosting supplements under a doctor's supervision and in combination with other treatments.

HIV AND OTHER INFECTIONS

HIV

Of all the horrors that come with HIV infection, one of the most tragically debilitating is the deterioration of the nervous system. To make things even worse, this aspect of the infection attacks children in particular. The brain damage seen in some HIV-infected patients resembles that found in children with defective folate metabolism and in adults with severe deficiencies of vitamin B_{12}.

All these similarities set some scientists to wondering if methyl-metabolism deficiencies might be involved in nervous system disorders related to HIV infection and AIDS. In the early 1990s one team of investigators decided to test the idea. The researchers measured several indicators of methyl metabolism in six young children (1½ to 3 years old) with congenital HIV infection and neurological problems. Five of these children had neurological symptoms, while one did not. But even the patient without neurological symptoms had white-matter lesions in the brain that spoke of damage to the myelin sheath. The scientists found that levels of SAM and methylfolate in the cerebrospinal fluid of these children were significantly lower than in normal children aged one to five years. Cerebrospinal fluid SAM was less than half the level found in normal children, while cerebrospinal fluid methylfolate was less than one-third the level found in normal children. Because of other studies linking methyl deficiency with demyelination and neurological deterioration, the researchers suggested that defective methylation was probably responsible for neurological deterioration in these HIV-infected children. The loss of SAM and methylfolate—and the accompanying disintegration of the myelin sheath—may have been caused by the HIV infection, or the three disorders may be linked in some as yet unknown way.

As we all know, in most cases infection with HIV eventually brings on AIDS. But that's not true of everyone who is HIV-positive. And even for the vast majority of infected people who do develop the disease, there can be a big difference in the lag time between infection and the appearance of AIDS symptoms. Some HIV-positive patients develop full-blown AIDS in a matter of months, while others remain healthy and free of symptoms for many years. This has long been one of the central mysteries in the ongoing story of the AIDS epidemic. Ten years ago a group of researchers set out to shed some light on this mystery by doing a long-term study of 310 HIV-positive males in the Baltimore and Washington, D.C., areas. Among the things the scientists looked at in this study were levels of specific nutrients. From the standpoint of methylation, the results were eye-opening. Those men in the study who had low blood serum levels of vitamin B_{12} developed AIDS more quickly (usually within four years) than those with higher B_{12} levels, many of whom went as long as eight years before the AIDS symptoms began to show up. However, low serum B_6 and folate levels were not associated with faster progression to the full-blown disease. These results turned out to be true no matter how old the patients were, what drugs they were taking, or even how much alcohol they drank.

There are other signposts that methylation is related to HIV infection. In 1996 scientists published a study in which they had looked at blood levels of HCY in twenty-one HIV-positive patients. The total concentration of HCY was normal. But when the scientists took a closer look, they found that levels of what is called "free" HCY (that is, HCY molecules that are not bound to any other molecules) was significantly higher in HIV-infected patients than in healthy people. At the same time, the researchers found that methionine was lower in the HIV-infected patients. Remember that low levels of methionine are another indication that methyl metabolism is lagging.

So it seems possible that a *Methyl Magic* program may help people who are HIV-positive stay healthy longer and may even stave off full-blown AIDS indefinitely. Remember, though, that patients should work with their doctors and not abandon other potentially worthwhile treatments while they're trying methyl-boosting supplements. Also, if the patient has cancer, he or she will be charting new territory by using methyl-boosting supplements and should do so only with extreme caution, medical advice, and supervision. Note that at this time I do *not* recommend methyl supplements for people with cancer.

OTHER INFECTIONS

HIV infection is by no means the only infectious disease in which changes in methyl metabolism may be an important factor. Three other examples are influenza, mono–nucleosis, and at least one type of pneumonia, known as *mycoplasma* pneumonia. Scientists have examined folate levels in patients suffering from all three of these infections. Again, the results are revealing. At least 50 percent of the flu patients had low levels of folate. The percentage of patients suffering from the other two infections who also had low folate levels was even higher: 60 percent and 73 percent, respectively. The researchers subsequently investigated chronic fatigue syndrome (CFS) because of a possible viral origin of this disease. The proportion of these CFS patients deficient in folate was 50 percent.

It may be that low folate predisposed these patients to get sick in the first place. On the other hand, the diseases themselves may have caused folate levels to drop. In either case, variations in folate levels could help explain the variations in time required for different people to fully recover from infection and could offer clues to why infections are often implicated in triggering CFS, MS, and other chronic diseases.

Once I began taking methyl supplements, I noticed that I got fewer colds. On the rare occasions when I do get a cold, it's usually less severe. Sometimes I'll feel just a little "off" for a few days, then notice a sniffle or two one or two days later. It's only after the cold is almost over that I notice it! A number of people have told me they've experienced the same healthy trend after they started taking methylating supplements. This is not hard science, but a number of these observations are intriguing and consistent with some of the scientific findings just discussed. This is clearly an area where more studies are needed.

UNDERLYING MECHANISMS OF DISEASE

When it comes right down to it, many (if not most) diseases start at the level of the cell. Methyl metabolism is clearly a vital cog in the machinery that makes cells function, grow, divide, and proliferate. So diseases in which cell proliferation has gone awry might be better understood when we know more about the details of the role of methyl metabolism in these basic cellular functions.

The list of such diseases is impressively long and includes many of our most common killers—cancer, for example, and arteriosclerosis. It also includes rheumatoid arthritis and some immune system disorders, and it may bear some relationship to ailments in which inflammation plays a part, such as lupus, rheumatoid arthritis, osteoarthritis, psoriasis, and asthma. These and other diseases may involve viral or bacterial infections. In those cases cell proliferation is also an important component. So it would be useful to know how methyl metabolism is related to inflammatory and infectious diseases in general and thus add to our knowledge of the pivotal role methyl metabolism plays in a wide variety of diseases.

GENERAL APPROACH TO DIAGNOSIS

Despite the obvious importance of methyl metabolism in human disease, the news has yet to make much of an impact where it's needed most—in the doctor's office. Few physicians run tests that include a full account of methyl metabolites. Plasma HCY, methionine loading, blood folate, B_{12}, MMA, blood SAM, white blood cell DNA methylation, cerebrospinal fluid HCY, SAM, folate, B_{12}, and others can all be useful in diagnosis. At the same time, we need to take a closer look at the possibility that "normal" levels of these methylating nutrients may not be adequate to prevent or treat disease. Such testing is important not only for getting at the cause of disease, but also because, as we've said so often, most deficiencies in methyl metabolism can be treated easily and effectively by diet and dietary supplements. In cases where a disease is caused by nutritional deficiency—especially by deficiencies in methylating nutrients—it is tragic when patients are not treated appropriately. Many of these patients probably suffer or even die from a seemingly intractable disease simply because their deficiency hasn't been identified.

CHAPTER 14

METHYL MAGIC AND THE MIND

Even if we knew nothing about how Methyl Magic supplements affect mood or memory, we would suspect that methylation would have an important impact on how we feel, think, and remember. Why? Because we know that methylation is a critical aid in the metabolism of most neurotransmitters, the vital substances that carry the brain's messages. Methylation is also required for the maintainence of our myelin, the material that insulates our nerve fibers and helps transmit the nervous system's signals. You'll recall that loss of myelin causes, or is accompanied by, MS and a variety of severe neurological disorders. It turns out that demyelination is also implicated in a wide range of psychiatric ailments, including some cases of schizophrenia and depression.

If methylation deficiencies are involved in these mental illnesses, can correcting the deficiencies by using methyl-boosting supplements help treat the diseases? The answer may well be "yes." For example, a number of studies show that 10 to 50 percent of psychiatric patients have low folate levels and many have low vitamin B_{12} levels. Other studies reveal that many depressed people are methyl deficient by one criterion or another and that correction of this deficiency can eliminate depression. Some very encouraging studies also suggest that methyl supplements may help relieve schizophrenia.

SAM performs so many functions in neurotransmitter metabolism and other processes in our brains that SAM's actions relating to our mood and perception are probably multifold. These include the following:

1. SAM makes melatonin out of N-acetylserotonin, and melatonin helps regulate our sleep cycles.
2. SAM makes adrenaline, an important stimulant, from noradrenaline.
3. SAM aids in the turnover (clearance) of histamine. Without SAM, histamine would accumulate, causing allergic and inflammatory responses. In the brain histamine is also a neurotransmitter.
4. SAM assists in the turnover (clearance) of dopamine, which is a very important mood regulator.
5. SAM makes acetylcholine, vital to memory, cognition (especially as we get older), energy, the development of embryonic brains, and the maintenance of adult brains.
6. SAM keeps cell membranes fluid by making phosphatidylcholine. Loss of membrane fluidity is associated with aging, so keeping membranes fluid may help preserve the normal functions of our cells. Maintaining membrane fluidity may even help slow the aging process.

Because SAM has so many functions, a shortfall in SAM can contribute to a number of mental and emotional disorders.

DEPRESSION

Clinical depression is strongly correlated with dietary methyl deficiency. Low blood folates, low vitamin B_{12}, low blood SAM, and high HCY have all been associated with clinical depression. Many researchers look on SAM and other key constituents of methyl metabolism, such as folic acid, as an important regulator of moods. As such, these methyl-boosting substances can have a strong impact on treating even severe cases of depression.

Even used alone, with no other methylating supplements, SAM is an effective antidepressant. In 1990 a group of scientists led by Dr. Bruce L. Kagan, Psychiatric and Behavioral Sciences, UCLA, set out to prove this connection. They enrolled eighteen inpatients who met the *Diagnostic and Statistical Manual of Mental Disorders* (*DSM-III*) criteria for major depression. These patients were randomly assigned to receive either 200 milligrams oral SAM tablets or placebo tablets identical in appearance. Some patients were gradually given increased doses of SAM or the placebo for the first week, but most were given 800 milligrams SAM or the placebo twice a day (total of 1,600 milligrams per day) for each of twenty-one days. Patients were rated for depression on the first day of the study, then four more times over three weeks.

Of the fifteen patients finishing the study, test scores showed that the SAM group had significantly reduced depression compared with the placebo group. The SAM group showed response in just seven days and were still improving at the end of the twenty-one-day trial. The Kagan study is just one of the many trials that have shown conclusively that SAM works better than placebos in treating depression.

It may not come as a big surprise that SAM is a better antidepressant than sugar pills. Perhaps even more important are studies that show that SAM works at least as well as a number of common antidepressant drugs, including imipramine and desipramine. One study comparing imipramine with SAM found that more patients improved when using SAM than when using the antidepressant drug. An interesting and surprising side: Concentrations of SAM in the blood increased in the patients with the greatest improvement, whether they were treated with SAM or with imipramine. SAM was not only effective, it was safe, showing no long-term or serious side effects. The only exception noted in Kagan's study was one patient who became manic. Other researchers have shown that SAM can trigger a manic episode. Consequently SAM is not recommended for treatment of manic-depression.

Kagan's study was one of many to evaluate SAM's potential as an antidepressant. In 1994 scientists took a combined look at thirteen of these studies, involving about four hundred patients. In these selected studies researchers used at least 200 milligrams per day of SAM intravenously or at least 1,600 milligrams per day of SAM orally. As in Kagan's study, the results showed that SAM was an effective antidepressant compared with a placebo and that it was as effective as several other antidepressants.

These trials confirmed the view of the medical community in Europe, where SAM tablets are often used as an antidepressant, with good to excellent results. SAM has some important advantages over antidepressant drugs. SAM gives a more rapid response, often showing results in just a few days. SAM has very few side effects; these are generally mild—nausea, restlessness, and minor anxiety—and confined to a small number of patients.

SAM is by no means the only methyl booster that can help treat depression. Folates have a good record as well. Clinical studies have shown that depression correlates most strongly with low blood folate levels. Folic acid and methylfolate have been used as antidepressants alone or in combination with other antidepressants. In fact, folic acid has even been used in combination with lithium to improve treatment of manic depression.

In one especially revealing study, researchers enrolled 213 patients in an eight-week trial of fluoxetine (the active ingredient of Prozac). Every two weeks the patients were rated for depression. At the same time, scientists checked the patients' blood serum for markers of methyl metabolism—not only for folate, but also for vitamin B_{12} and HCY. Levels of one or more of these markers were abnormal in 36 percent of patients. Low folate levels in particular were significantly associated with melancholic depression and with lack of response to treatment with fluoxetine. Other studies indicated that geriatric patients with low folate levels responded less well to such antidepressants as sertraline or nortriptyline.

If we look at them as a whole, these numerous studies show convincingly that SAM is an effective antidepressant and that some other methyl supplements—folates in particular—can in at least some cases help treat depression. Heart patients treated with betaine have reported lasting improvement in their sense of well-being with some remarking that they never felt so good. Studies of a wide variety of antidepressants show that SAM and folate are important in the regulation of mood and in the outcome of antidepressant treatment. The bottom line is these many findings confirm the general relationship between methylation and mood.

A number of these and other studies indicate that keeping folic acid levels in the high end of the normal range or higher will help minimize depression. Even depressed patients whose folate is "normal" can be helped by supplements of this methyl booster.

If SAM and folate can help relieve depression, can these and other methyl supplements be useful in treating not only depression, but a wide variety of mental disorders? Here again, the answer seems to be "yes." In 1988 scientists at the Columbia-Presbyterian Medical and Harlem Hospital Centers in New York City reported the results of a large, seventeen-year study of vitamin B_{12} deficiency in 141 patients who were suffering from neuropsychiatric disorders, including depression, memory loss, agitation, hallucinations, fatigue, sensory losses, abnormal gait, and weakness in the arms and legs. Besides vitamin B_{12} deficiency, the researchers found another telltale sign of methylation problems. Among the patients in the study who were tested for HCY, nearly all had high HCY levels—even if the rest of their blood tests (other than vitamin B_{12}) were normal.

When the researchers gave these patients injections of vitamin B_{12}, all but one (a patient who died) showed general improvement in their neuropsychiatric disorders. In fact, many of them became entirely free of neurological symptoms as long as they remained on B_{12} therapy. This is truly an amazing result. It's rare in medical science that a single, simple treatment has such a powerful and widespread impact in such an astonishingly high percentage of patients. This demonstrates the power and effectiveness of measuring the blood for nutrients first, so that these conditions can be properly diagnosed and nutritional treatments used effectively.

The evidence that low folate, low B_{12}, low SAM, or high HCY are causes or risk factors for depression or psychiatric disorders is all but overwhelming. So it makes sense for doctors and psychiatrists to take these factors into account when they treat these ailments. Thus low folate, low B_{12}, and high HCY are easy to correct with proper diet and *Methyl Magic* supplements. Low levels of SAM can probably also be treated by this same kind of nutritional intervention, but we have less data to clinch the case. Certainly low blood SAM is treatable with intravenous or even oral SAM.

We still don't know exactly why SAM or folates work so well as antidepressants or why betaine would improve one's sense of well-being. Folates and betaine probably act through the production of SAM, and SAM is centrally involved in the metabolism of many neurotransmitters. It helps metabolize, transport, and clear both dopamine and serotonin. Transit of dopamine and serotonin is considered important in the regulation of mood. Excesses of these vital messenger chemicals may be involved, for example, in schizophrenia and manic-depression. Also, SAM is needed to make choline and, in turn, the neurotransmitter acetylcholine. Because choline also effects mood and memory, increases in acetylcholine are a likely explanation for some of SAM's beneficial effects.

The conclusion is all but inescapable: First of all, deficits in methylating nutrients—and high levels of HCY—are correlated with, if not sometimes a cause of, a variety of psychiatric disorders. Second, factors that improve methyl metabolism—the now familiar methyl boosters such as folic acid, SAM, vitamin B_{12}, betaine, and choline—also often improve mood, memory, and alertness.

SCHIZOPHRENIA

Many people, influenced by inaccurate novels and movies, think of schizophrenia as the "split personality" disease. Actually schizophrenia has nothing to do with split or multiple personalities. Rather, it's, as *Webster's Medical Dictionary* defines it, "a psychotic disorder characterized by loss of contact with the environment, by noticeable deterioration in the level of functioning in everyday life, and by disintegration of the personality. . . ." Victims of schizophrenia often experience delusions and hallucinations, many of which can be truly terrifying.

Schizophrenia illustrates an important point about methylation and methylation research. Scientists have long suspected that methylation has a role in schizophrenia. This suspicion led a number of researchers to treat victims of schizophrenia with methionine, the assumption being that increases in methionine would increase methylation. The amounts of methionine given schizophrenics in these studies was usually between 5 and 40 grams per day. This is a very substantial amount of methionine—probably two to twenty times what someone might get in a normal diet. Most of these patients experienced a deterioration in their condition and an increase in psychosis, including, in over one-third of the patients, an increase in auditory and visual hallucinations or delusions. Less than 10 percent of the patients showed improvement.

The ironic truth, which was not appreciated until later, is that high doses of methionine alone increase HCY. You'll recall that high levels of HCY are a sign of methylation deficiency. Subsequent studies have shown that large doses of methionine can put even normal, healthy people on a "methyl roller coaster," in which both HCY and SAM rise and fall precipitously during the course of a day. This methyl roller-coaster ride could well have noticeable effects on schizophrenics.

HCY, METHYL MAGIC, AND SCHIZOPHRENIA

During the mid-1970s, a fifteen-year-old girl was admitted to Johns Hopkins Hospital in Baltimore. To put it mildly, the girl was in bad shape. From the age of twelve she had experienced trouble concentrating and doing activities she had once done well. She forgot how to tell time, to read, and to do schoolwork. Over the next three years her condition deteriorated so markedly that psychiatrists eventually diagnosed her condition as catatonic schizophrenia. By the time she entered the hospital she was nearly mute, withdrawn, and experiencing hallucinations. To make things even worse, she suffered a seizure, leading doctors to suspect that she had a degenerative disease of the central nervous system.

After a battery of tests, blood and urine analyses showed that the girl's HCY level was so high that she had homocystinuria. Her doctors immediately started her on methylating therapy, giving her first vitamin B_6 and later folic acid. Soon her HCY level declined dramatically, and her condition improved noticeably. Although she still showed signs of nervous system disease, her symptoms of schizophrenia all but disappeared.

Sound like a happy ending? Well, not yet. Several months later she returned to the hospital, suffering symptoms similar to her pretreatment condition. This time doctors tested her for an enzyme called *methylenetetrahydrofolate reductase* (*MTHFR*), an essential enzyme in the methylation of folate. She was found deficient in this enzyme, so doctors again gave her folic acid. As before, her condition improved substantially. Thus supplemental folic acid was clearly effective in treating and eliminating this patient's psychotic condition.

As it turns out, a number of studies now show that HCY levels are elevated in schizophrenics. At the same time, deficiencies in folate seem to be related to this terrifying mental disease. In 1990 researchers tested 123 psychiatric patients for red cell folate and found one-third (41 patients) to be clearly folate deficient or borderline deficient. Of these, scientists chose 17 schizophrenics (along with 24 depressed patients) for further study. About half the patients were given 15 milligrams of methylfolate every day for six months. The other half got only a placebo.

Both groups—schizophrenics and depressed patients—who took the methylfolate showed gradual improvement. After three months folates in the blood serum and the red blood cells were much improved in the patients who had taken methylfolate. Those who got only the placebo showed little or no improvement. For those in the methylfolate groups, improvement in folate levels continued to the sixth month of the study. Boosting folate levels had a significant effect on the patients' mental illness. After three months the rating score of the methylfolate-treated depressed patients was markedly improved. After six months both depressed patients and schizophrenic patients had shown significant psychiatric improvement.

The lesson to be learned here is that it is important to distinguish nutritional deficiencies—especially those involving methylation—in schizophrenia, as well as in other psychiatric disorders. While it's unlikely that nutriton alone will cure most schizophrenics, a combination of methylation therapy with antipsychotic drugs may be an effective treatment for many.

CHOLINE, MEMORY, AND MENTAL FUNCTION

Choline and its relative, the neurotransmitter acetylcholine, are crucial "lubricants" that help keep our mental machinery running smoothly. Study after study has shown that choline improves memory in humans—both the old and the young. In fact, in some of these experiments people who appear to have the poorest memories have shown the most improvement!

Why is this so? Again, methylation is a vital key. The brain cells known as *neurons* have a tremendous appetite for choline, which they use to help send chemical signals to other neurons. These cells get their choline by "harvesting" it from the blood. Choline comes from the diet or is made by the liver. When the liver makes choline it starts the process by using three molecules of SAM to methylate a substance called *phosphatidylethanolamine*. This substance is then transformed to *phosphatidycholine* (*PC*), which in turn releases the choline that the neurons and other cells use for "food" to make acetylcholine for communicating with their neighbor neurons. To satiate its appetite for choline, the brain uses a *lot* of choline methyl groups, and a lot of SAM.

So how do we replenish these methylators and keep the brain's appetite satisfied? Well, there's a significant amount of choline in coffee. Research with rats shows that a combination of caffeine and choline releases much more acetylcholine than choline alone. Yet caffeine by itself didn't increase acetylcholine, either. So in this study, at least, it was the combination of caffeine and choline that did the trick.

But you don't have to resort to caffeine, which if taken in excess can create other health problems, to keep your brain well fed with choline and acetylcholine. *Methyl Magic* can do the job. I've experienced this mental alertness personally, using overall methyl supplementation as described in chapter 5, and also by using either choline or betaine alone. Before I started my *Methyl Magic* program, by four P.M. on most afternoons I got hit with "brain drain." Since I've embarked on my personal methylation experiment I have been much more alert, so much so that I've been able to blast right through that four o'clock slump. I hear the same happy reports from other people who are using methyl-boosting supplements, many of whom tell me that their memory has improved as well. So here's a case where science and anecdote point in exactly the same direction: the power of *Methyl Magic* can rev up your brain and even shore up a sagging memory.

ALZHEIMER'S DISEASE

By now most of us are familiar with the ravages of Alzheimer's disease—the gradual loss of memory, starting with seemingly innocuous lapses, then progressing slowly until victims cannot remember who they are or where they live or even recognize their loved ones. Perhaps you've had a relative, even a parent, with the disease and have seen firsthand how it can reduce a once alert person to a state of tragic helplessness. Ultimately, of course, the disease can kill. To those who have suffered through the long period of disintegration, or watched others suffer through it, death can seem a final kindness.

There are any number of theories as to what might cause Alzheimer's—unfortunate genes, infections by viruses, formation of destructive plaques in the brain, and inflammation, among others. But no matter which of these causes, or combinations of them, ultimately proves correct, there's little doubt that methylation plays a part in the disease, and there's hope that methyl-boosting supplements can be of at least some help in treating it.

Knowing what we do about the role of choline in memory, it's not surprising that this methylating nutrient has long been associated with Alzheimer's. In fact, choline in various forms has had some impact on treating the disease, at least in terms of slowing its progress. One of those forms, of course, is choline itself. In the past sometimes large amounts of choline, such as 10 grams a day, have been given to Alzheimer's patients. This was not a popular treatment with patients' families or caregivers, because breakdown of choline can produce a substance called *trimethylamine,* which often leaves patients smelling fishy. In smaller doses—(1 to 2 grams of choline a day)—this fishy smell can be eliminated by taking 800 micrograms of folic acid at the same time. It has not yet been determined if this tactic works with choline doses as large as 10 grams a day.

Lecithin, also known as phosphatidylcholine (PC), is another form of choline that's been used in attempts to slow progression of the disease. Some people prefer it because it doesn't produce the fishy smell associated with large doses of choline. But lecithin contains only a small amount of choline, so it's not a very efficient source of this methylating nutrient.

One source of choline that shows some promise is a compound called *cytidine 5'-diphosphocholine* (*CDP-choline*). Taken orally, CDP-choline is well absorbed by the body, and its choline content is readily taken up by the brain. Like choline itself, CDP-choline affects neurotransmitter levels and contributes to the synthesis of PC. CDP-choline has been reported to slow the progression of Alzheimer's in some patients. These results may also be true of SAM, and may turn out to be true of betaine as well.

Recent studies clearly show that high HCY, low folate, and low vitamin B_{12} accompany, and may help bring on, Alzheimer's disease. Again this is just one more reason to consider methylating supplements for prevention and slowing of Alzheimer's. Because of the severe memory and nerve cell loss in Alzheimer's, other treatments that will hopefully be available in the future, such as those to regenerate neurons, will probably be the best bet. In the meantime, methylating supplements may help prevent or postpone Alzheimer's.

There's little doubt that methylation is involved in a number of serious mental disorders. It may well be that boosting methylation with *Methyl Magic* supplements will help tame these diseases and at least partially relieve the suffering that accompanies them.

CHAPTER 15

AGING AND LONGEVITY

*The reasons for some animals being long-lived and
others short-lived and, in a word,
causes of the length and brevity of life call for investigation.*

Aristotle, 350 B.C. *"On Longevity
and Shortness of Life,"
as translated by G.R.T. Ross*

From the time I was five, the mysteries of aging and longevity drew me toward science and biology. If I could help solve, or at least shed some light on, these mysteries, it might help alleviate the suffering and deterioration associated with growing older, and it might help us live out what many experts think is our allotted healthy life span of 120 years or more. Indeed, much of this book has focused on diseases that are to a large degree age related. Early in my career as a scientist I became convinced that regulating methylation in our bodies was one of the keys to aging gracefully and living long and healthy lives. I remain convinced today.

HCY, FOLATES, AGING, AND LONGEVITY

As we've shown, it is likely that HCY in unhealthy excess causes vascular disease—arteriosclerosis and thrombosis—which can lead to heart attack and stroke. But what does "unhealthy excess" mean? To answer that question, we need to look at what the medical community considers "normal" levels of HCY. The consensus among doctors and scientists is that the "normal" level for HCY in blood plasma is about 10 micromolar. After all, we all need some amount of HCY in our blood, in that HCY is an essential component of methyl metabolism. The question to ask is: What level of HCY is safe? An even better question: For preserving health, preventing disease, and extending longevity, what level of HCY is *optimal*?

That's a tough question. But fortunately we have some clues. Premenopausal women have relatively little vascular disease. Among adults, younger women also have some of the lowest levels of HCY. If we were to focus a large-scale scientific effort on studying these women—or studying any group of people with low HCY—it might help us get a better idea of what levels are optimal. In the meantime, I propose that the "normal" levels of HCY (that is, around 10 micromolar) are too high and that they contribute to aging and age-related disease. In some people HCY is at levels of 4 to 6 micromolar. This is probably as safe as, if not safer than, levels of 8, 10, or 12 micromolar. At this point we can estimate, but we really don't know. One place to start is to survey HCY in the healthiest, most disease-free groups of people and work from there.

Most people seem worried about heart attack and stroke. It is said that if you could prevent heart disease, you might add several years to the average life span. But what goes into the calculation for determining average life span? Probably just the major diseases—heart attack and stroke. These calculations often don't take into account so-called lesser but still dangerous related diseases such as claudication and peripheral vascular disease.

Maybe there's more to all this than a first glance reveals. Why do we find HCY in the blood in the first place? Well, it's there at least in part because of cells that can't process it fast enough and have to "export" it. The cells send HCY out through the cell membrane into the fluid between cells that basically becomes, or is, the blood plasma. It's a lot like putting the trash from inside your house through the door and out onto the curb for pickup. You figure it'll be picked up and taken somewhere to be recycled or degraded and you'll buy some new stuff to replace it. Well, if cells could think, they'd probably come to the same conclusion. Let's just put HCY out on the curb, let the blood take it, and the liver will recycle it. That's what we pay the liver to do, right? That will keep us (the cells) from accumulating a bunch of junk we'll never use, or even toxic waste, which is what excess HCY amounts to.

But what if the junk that's meant to be recycled—the excess HCY—doesn't get taken out to the curb? Or even if it does, what if the "garbage truck"—the bloodstream—doesn't haul off the HCY far enough or fast enough? Think about what happens during a big city garbage strike. First the sidewalks get choked with untransported trash. Theoretically if the sidewalks get completely clogged, people can't get out of their houses to go shopping. The result? They starve to death. A version of the same thing happens in your body. If HCY isn't hauled away, chances are that, first, your smallest blood vessels—veins, capillaries, and tiny arteries called *arterioles*—will develop arteriosclerosis and start to clog up. What happens next? The cells go right on exporting HCY to the blood plasma. If your circulation is poor because your small blood vessels are narrowed and partially clogged, HCY could build up to higher levels because it's less quickly and less efficiently moved out to the liver. I suspect that, just as in a garbage strike, HCY buildup causes worse arteriosclerosis, more narrowing and clogging, and that this leads to even more HCY buildup. Sound like a vicious circle?

So next along this vicious circle, small, usually microscopic, sections of your body (groups of cells) would eventually die off by "suffocating"—or by choking on their own excess garbage. What if this happened over time throughout your body? You'd slowly shrivel and die. Sound like the aging process? We don't know whether or not HCY contributes to aging by choking off small blood vessels in this way. But it seems logical. A major tip-off is that it's been shown that the highest risk for vascular disease as a result of elevated HCY is from vascular disease in the small, or *peripheral,* blood vessels.

So let's say for the moment that so-called normal levels of HCY are actually unhealthy and can cause a whole range of potentially debilitating and even deadly problems. Well, the HCY story actually gets worse. HCY levels, which may be too high even when we're in our thirties (or might be too high in our small blood vessels), actually tend to get higher with age.

A number of studies over recent years have shown this to be true. One of them, conducted in Sweden, looked at HCY and a series of other factors in 244 men and women aged 35 to 95. The results showed that blood plasma HCY definitely rose with age. If you look at the graph presented here, you'll see that by the ages of 80 and 90 HCY levels have risen steeply. If the same pattern continued, by the age of 120 all these people who already have hyperhomocysteinemia would be likely to have homocystinuria. While such an extrapolation may be a bit of a stretch, the curve is definitely headed up. It could be that HCY is one thing that limits our life span to the often assumed limit of 120 years.

HOMOCYSTINURIA: CLUES TO AGING

In many ways, homocystinuria, the disease that's defined by extremely high levels of HCY, looks a great deal like premature aging. People who suffer from homocystinuria can fall prey to a wide range of ailments or conditions that are usually thought to be age related—everything from serious vascular and nervous system disorders to graying hair and "aging" skin. These intriguing similarities may help shed light on the relationship between aging and methylation.

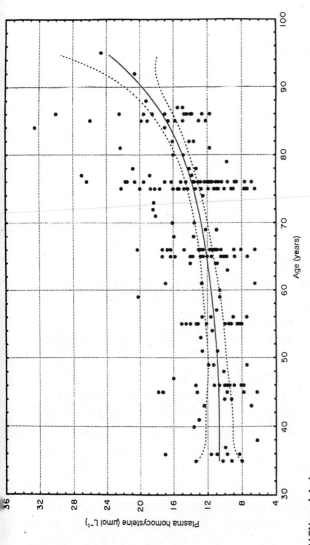

Plasma HCY and Aging

Plasma HCY tracked with age. The solid line represents the average HCY levels from the 244 people in the study. The dotted lines on either side of the solid line represent statistical variance of the figures represented by the solid line. Reproduced from Brattstrom, L., Lindgren, A., Israelsson, B., Andersson, A., and Hultberg, B. (1994). Homocysteine and cysteine: determinants of plasma levels in middle-aged and elderly subjects. *Journal of Internal Medicine* 236, 633–41, with permission.

We've already had a look at the role HCY plays in the development of vascular disease and disorders of the nervous system. Now let's turn our attention to another ailment, which can be a feature of either homocystinuria or "normal" aging. That condition is *osteoporosis*, a loss of bone mass and density that makes the bones fragile and the victim more vulnerable to fractures. Some doctors refer to osteoporosis as the "brittle bone disease." A number of researchers have suggested that moderately high HCY—in the 15 to 30 micromolar range—may play a role in causing osteoporosis.

Homocystinurics often have very serious osteoporosis, tendency to fracture, and *scoliosis*—an abnormal curvature of the spine. One report studied twenty-six homocystinureics between six and forty-five years of age. The results are consistent with those of surveys reported by others. All but one of the patients had osteoporotic vertebrae, while seventeen had scoliosis and five had exaggerated thoracic kyphosis ("hunchback"). Other symptoms included calcific spicules in the joints, a variety of spinal deformities, degeneration of intervertebral disks, chronic back pain, and large knobby knees. The risk of developing these often debilitating disorders as we get older is just one more reason to keep HCY low by means of a *Methyl Magic* program.

Another affliction that can be an aspect of either homocystinuria or "normal" aging is cataracts. Cataracts are caused in part by oxidative damage and photo damage to the eye lens, but low methylation is also thought to play a role in the development of this disease, which can lead to partial or complete blindness. In this affliction an enzyme called *protein L-isoaspartyl methyltransferase (PIMT)*, which repairs age-related protein damage, is important. Specific kinds of protein damage are found in the eye lenses of people who suffer from cataracts. One study has shown that the gene for the protein repair enzyme PIMT is expressed far less in the lenses of cataract patients than in those of people with normal vision.

What does this have to do with methylation? Well, when eye lens proteins are damaged, PIMT uses SAM to methylate these wayward proteins and bring them back to their normal state. While this doesn't necessarily tell us the role of methyl metabolism in cataract formation, it may tell us that this type of protein damage is increased in cataracts and may contribute to their formation. It certainly suggests that methyl metabolism may be important, because we know from other cases that when SAM is less available, or when levels of its cousin, SAH, are elevated, methylation reactions can be inhibited.

While far from a crippling disease, graying hair is certainly a hallmark of advancing age. Prematurely gray hair (or, in some cases, abnormally light hair) is also a common feature of homocystinuria. The hair of homocystinurics can also be unattractively coarse and brittle. For people with homocystinuria it's bad enough to have to battle the serious ravages of the disease, but even worse when one feels the ailment is robbing them of their youthful look.

But there are hints that *Methyl Magic* might help make hair healthier. At least one patient with the light hair characteristic of homocystinuria began to grow new, dark, and softer hair after vitamin B_6 therapy. Apparently, lowering HCY restored her natural hair color. Similar experiences have been reported in homocystinuria patients whose hair had gone prematurely gray. Again, lowering HCY through methylating supplements brought back youthful dark hair. If people with homocystinuria can "turn back the clock" this way by taking methylating supplements, can the "normal" graying that accompanies aging be reversed in the same way? We don't know yet, but it's certainly an intriguing possibility.

As if all these unfortunate effects of homocystinuria weren't bad enough, the disease can also affect the skin, making it thin and translucent, causing loss of skin pigmentation and mottled skin color. In at least one patient skin became coarse and inflexible. This patient's skin became more soft and pliable after therapy with methylating nutrients. If this is true for people with homocystinuria, we might speculate that in normal people, keeping HCY low, rather than slightly elevated, will help maintain soft, pliable skin. That possibility is certainly worth a closer look.

If HCY levels rise with age, we would suspect that methylating nutrients like vitamin B_{12} and folate would be decreasing. Well, the Swedish study mentioned previously did indeed show that HCY was higher when blood levels of folate or B_{12} were lower. But as folate and B_{12} increased *within the normal range*, HCY levels dropped. In fact, some of the people in the study group had high HCY even though the levels of B_{12} and folate, in both diet and bloodstream, were "normal." In these cases, apparently, the body was not using these methyl-boosting nutrients efficiently. This is a strong indication that so-called normal levels of folate and B_{12} are not necessarily enough to keep HCY levels in check.

In the Swedish study, those people who reported that they regularly took multivitamins had significantly lower HCY—3 micromolar less than people who didn't take multivitamins. This is another strong argument for the vitamin supplementation in the *Methyl Magic* program. The elderly should have their HCY monitored on a regular basis—at least once a year and more often if they want to test whether or not methylating supplements are in fact controlling their HCY levels. Many people will probably find that extra nutritional support is needed to keep HCY low.

By following these recommendations, HCY can be reduced to very low levels in the elderly, even though the level may start out elevated. For example, in one study reported in the journal *Lancet* in 1995, scientists gave a group of elderly patients (aged seventy-two to eighty) with HCY in the 11 to 14 micromolar range injections of 1 milligram vitamin B_{12}, 1.1 milligrams folic acid, and 5 milligrams vitamin B_6 for each of several days over three weeks. In this group the average HCY level dropped to 8 micromolar. This is even lower than the "normal" level (~10.5 micromolar) for healthy thirty-five-year-olds!

Of course, vascular disease, deteriorating bones and skin, and so forth, are only some of the denizens that accompany aging. As we grow older we're more subject to mood disorders like depression. Our memories begin to slip, we're less alert, and we're more likely to be dependent on others for care. All these hallmarks of age-related deterioration seem to be linked to elevated HCY and/or low folate levels. Numerous researchers have reported such findings. In one recent study researchers looked at folate intake and serum and red blood cell folate in 177 healthy, independently living, elderly people aged sixty-five to eighty-nine years. At the same time, the scientists assessed the subjects' self-sufficiency—ability to perform household chores, shop, use the telephone, use transportation, handle finances, and take medication. The scientists also checked the volunteers for moderate mental deterioration.

The results were intriguing. Those subjects with adequate scores on mental state exams and independent living exams had significantly higher folate levels than those who had scored poorly. At the same time—and this finding has been replicated in many other studies—those subjects with low folate were significantly more likely to suffer from geriatric depression. While this team of scientists did not give folate supplements to their subjects, they refer to other researchers who have reported that simple correction of folate deficiency can transform some elderly people from being dependent and incapable to being independent and competent.

Obviously, then, older people who are still mentally healthy would be well advised to embark on the *Methyl Magic* program at the levels recommended in chapter 5. Certainly the time to address nutritional adequacy is before the onset of severe cognitive deterioration such as Alzheimer's disease. Even those already suffering from milder psychological disorders should find the *Methyl Magic* program beneficial.

It seems likely that as we age we have more at risk than our hearts, brains, and minds—as if those weren't enough! To maintain our appearance, our mental capacities, our fitness, and a satisfying sex life, we need clear blood vessels. So if we can keep HCY low and thus avoid the vicious circle of escalating HCY and escalating disease, we might do a great deal more than adding just several years to our lives. If we keep our methylation rates rolling along at a healthy clip, those extra years could be full of health, vitality, and joie de vivre. After all, most of us don't want to live longer if living longer means nothing more than added years of illness and infirmity. A good way to help prevent deterioration is to combine good nutrition with good circulation. The recipe? A healthy diet as described in chapter 4, regular exercise, and *Methyl Magic* supplementation.

CHOLINE AND THE AGING BRAIN

As we've seen, choline and one of its products, the neurotransmitter acetylcholine, are essential to the proper functioning of the brain. So it's important to ask what happens to these substances as we grow older. One team of scientists tackled this question in a study reported in the *Journal of the American Medical Association*. This team compared a group of physically and mentally healthy younger adults between the ages of twenty and forty years with a group of similarly healthy older adults aged sixty to eighty-five years. The scientists found that the younger people took much more choline into their brains from blood than did the older group. The researchers suggested that these differences in brain choline uptake may contribute to neurodegenerative, dementing illnesses such as senile dementia, or even Alzheimer's, that tend to strike late in life. They also suggested that older adults with higher levels of choline absorption may be at lower risk for dementias. These conclusions make sense, because in senile dementia and Alzheimer's, neurons that rely on choline show some of the most degeneration.

There's more to this story. Some scientists have proposed that when the brain runs short of acetylcholine, some of its cells try to make up the deficit by taking choline from their own membranes. (This process goes by the picturesque name of *autocannibalism*.) While this cannibalism may serve the short-term purpose of providing more acetylcholine for mental functioning, it may at the same time deplete neurons of essential components. Autocannibalism could also lead to lower membrane fluidity and altered enzyme activities in the membranes. Remember that membrane fluidity is vital to the healthy functioning of cells and that this fluidity tends to decline with age. On a chronic basis decreasing membrane fluidity could accelerate the aging process, especially in the areas of the brain that depend on choline. This could possibly even contribute to Alzheimer's disease.

The bottom line is that these studies, along with a number of others, suggest that the need for dietary choline appears to increase with age. Many nutritional recommendations for the elderly suggest choline intakes of 1 to 3 grams (1,000 to 3,000 milligrams) per day. I endorse these recommendations, but with the caution that people build up their choline intake gradually, over a month or so.

GENES, EVOLUTION, AND LONGEVITY

When people talk about aging and longevity, we often hear it said that "it's all in the genes." It seems nearly everyone has an uncle Fred or an aunt Margaret who smoked cigars, ate lard three times a day, and still made it to 106. Well, it's undeniably true that genetic differences among individuals have a great deal to do with health and longevity. In fact, these differences determine, at least in part, how long we live compared with others. As an example, people with homocystinuria do have genetic differences that can limit their life expectancy to only 2 to 20 years—even if they eat a "normal" diet. At the other, extreme end of the spectrum, a few lucky people on a "normal" diet make it to 120 years.

So genetic differences among human beings are powerful players in determining life expectancy. Gene differences among species are even more important. Species, from *Mus musculus* (the common mouse) to *Homo sapiens* (humans), evolved life spans and genes for longevity based on how long they typically survived in their natural environment. These genetic differences account for the fact that most common mice can live about 2 years, we humans live about 70 years, some tortoises live 150 years, and some trees live for thousands of years.

But even though all of us—from mice to men to bristlecone pine trees—evolved genes that determine our *maximum* life spans, these genes are getting hammered every day by our environment and even by our own inner workings. Now we have internal "mechanics" in place to repair the damage done by this hammering, but those mechanics aren't perfect. For one thing, the mechanics get their working orders from genes, which may themselves get damaged. Why aren't they perfect? Well, we evolved surrounded by everything from viruses, bacteria, and amoeba to lions, tigers, and bears trying to eat us. With all these natural enemies after us, we weren't likely to last more than forty years or so. So why would we evolve means to live two hundred years and perfect, invulnerable mechanics that would repair genetic damage effectively enough to ensure we lived that long?

Essentially evolution had a choice: given a certain level of ongoing damage, should we try to repair it all or repair just enough to get by for the few decades during which we have our babies? Evolution, in its blind wisdom, "decided" that it would be better to invest short term in more and better children. Thus we manage well enough to get by for a few decades. This leaves our genes still operating in the virus-, lion-, bacteria-, tiger-, amoeba-, and bear-threatened mode. So while we're busy building that "bridge to the twenty-first century," we're using largely Stone Age genes!

In human populations, as we've said, even these Stone Age genes vary greatly. This variation partly explains why we look and act differently from or similarly to others. Genetic variation also accounts for the fact that some people have high HCY on a "normal" diet, while others have "normal" HCY on a "normal" diet. It may also explain why some of us might respond to methyl deficiency by developing vascular disease, while others may respond by developing, say, a psychiatric disorder.

It's estimated that there are roughly one hundred thousand genes in the human genome—the genetic "map" of our species. At least a hundred (possibly double that number or more) of these genes are involved in methylation and methyl metabolism. Many of these genes provide "working orders" only for the enzymes involved in folate metabolism. Many others regulate the production of proteins that transport or bind vitamin B_{12}. In fact, there are probably at least one hundred methyltransferases that use SAM to donate methyl groups to another molecule, and each one has a gene all its own.

As in other areas of the human genome, variations in the genes that run our methyl machinery can have a huge impact on health. So some people may be genetically predisposed to high HCY, or low SAM, or inefficient use of folates, while in others those methylating functions may be fine. These differences in genome can draw the line between health and disease and perhaps even determine how well we age and how long we live.

Still, when all is said and done genetics is only one of the factors that affect methylation. Taken alone, genetics will not determine, say, an individual's HCY levels or one's susceptibility to disease. Remember that even in homocystinuria—among the most extreme cases of methylation disorders—HCY levels can be substantially reduced and the health of patients dramatically improved by specific methyl-boosting nutrients. In other words, moderate genetic susceptibilities and elevated HCY can certainly be controlled by a well-)designed program of diet and dietary supplements.

Entire cultures are able to avoid high levels of heart disease mainly by eating a different diet. For example, a traditional Japanese diet with fish, soybean, rice, and vegetables or a traditional Greek diet with olive oil instead of butter both aid in lowering occurrence of heart disease. Do these diets have an impact on improved methylation, lower HCY, and reduced incidence of age-related heart disease? Apparently so. One study compared the correlation between HCY levels and death from heart disease in several industrialized countries. In Spain, France, and Japan, with their "heart-healthy" diets, HCY levels averaged between 7 and 8 micromolar, and the incidence of death from heart disease was about 200 per 100,000 population every year. In Finland, on the other hand, where the diet is more like that in the United States, HCY averaged about 11 micromolar, and deaths from heart disease were about 500 per 100,000 population. In other words, a *difference* of only 3 to 4 micromolar in HCY meant death rates from heart disease 150 percent higher (2.5 times as high) in Finland than in the countries with healthier diets.

So greatly reducing heart disease and stroke incidence simply involves making some good choices about our diets and lifestyles. You can allow yourself to be a victim of your genetics and just let disease happen, or you can choose to take at least a measure of control over your health by following the *Methyl Magic* program.

AGING CELLS AND DNA METHYLATION

Nearly forty years ago Dr. Leonard Hayflick, now a University of California biologist and author of the recent book *How and Why We Age*, asked a very basic question about aging. We know that animals and tissues age, but do cells themselves age if separated from the whole animal or tissue? Some yeast and bacteria cells seem to go on living and reproducing indefinitely—would human cells do the same?

To answer the question, Hayflick put human connective tissue cells known as *fibroblasts* in test tubes and kept them bathed in a nutrient broth to keep them growing and dividing. Then he kept track of their numbers, tallying how many times they doubled. After fifty or so doublings, the cells stopped growing and eventually died. Although the number of doublings vary from one cell type to another, Hayflick and his coworkers eventually found that what was true for fibroblasts was also true for most types of cells—in mammals, at least.

This told him that human cells, like humans themselves, are not immortal. Many cancer cells, by the way, are an exception, in that they do keep growing and dividing indefinitely. Like our bodies, our cells do age and die. In fact, we now know that our cells and those of other mammals often show a variety of changes as they age. These include reduced ability to grow and divide and numerous cell dysfunctions. Sometimes these dysfunctions involve changes in a few genes, sometimes they involve actual conversion of the cell from one type to another. In one of the most extreme changes, the cells grow more rapidly than normal. If this growth remains uncontrolled, benign tumors or even cancer can result.

Except for tumor cells, most of the cells in our bodies age and eventually die. The big question, of course, is: What makes cells age? While a number of factors may contribute to cellular aging, one of the more likely is a gradual loss of DNA methylation. Experiments have shown that normal mammalian cells grown in culture dishes in the laboratory lose DNA methylation the more they grow and divide.

Does this mean that there's a link between cellular aging and decreases in overall DNA methylation? Apparently so. In fact, this link has been seen in a wide variety of animal tissues and organs. Dr. Boris Vanyushin and co-workers in Moscow first showed in the 1960s and published in 1967 that salmon lost DNA methylation with age. The same group of scientists later showed that what was true in salmon was also true for most of the organs they studied in cattle and rats. Later studies by several groups of scientists in the United States and Japan indicated that many organs in mice also showed loss of DNA methylation with aging.

But would this hold true for humans? The answer seems to be yes for some cell types, maybe no for others. For example, in humans, DNA methylation is lost with age in some types of immune system cells (lymphocytes and T-cells), in spleen cells, and in cells that line the bronchial tubes. In the liver, however, aging seems to bring no significant change in DNA methylation.

Still, in the big picture most organs and tissues of animals show DNA methylation losses with age. Interestingly enough, though, it seems that in general the longer an animal species' life span or the greater the doubling potential of a cell type, the better the species is able to maintain its DNA methylation. Many studies show that the maintenance of methylation is correlated with life span and may in fact be one mechanism for determining how long some animal species—including humans—live.

For example, in a landmark study, a team of scientists

at the National Cancer Institute and National Institutes of Aging, studied two subspecies of mice. One of these varieties, *Peromyscus leucopus*, the white-footed mouse, maintains DNA methylation approximately twice as well and has about twice the life span (average approximately four years, maximum about eight) as does *Mus*, the common house/laboratory mouse, which lives an average of two years. In the same study the researchers also compared human bronchial epithelial cells from donors of different ages. Their study showed that DNA methylation does decrease with age, but that DNA methylation was maintained much better in humans than in either type of mouse. They estimated that humans lost DNA methylation at less than one-tenth the rate of white-footed mice and at less than one-twentieth the rate of common house mice. These are only estimates because the experiments with humans and mice cannot be done in quite the same way. However, the two species of mice can be compared directly, and overall these results show a very close relationship between the rate of DNA methylation loss and life span. In this and other experiments, humans maintained their DNA methylation much better than the mice and, of course, lived much longer than any type of mouse.

To scientists this was fascinating news. It raised the possibility that by tinkering with DNA methylation in the laboratory, we might be able to alter the life span of human cells. We now know that this works in at least one direction. Short treatments with substances that inhibit DNA methylation significantly decrease the doubling potential of normal human fibroblast cells.

Because I knew that DNA methylation was dependent on methyl metabolism, I proposed that one reason we lose methylation with age is that our metabolisms were inadequate to the task of maintaining our DNA methylation. I proposed that most of our cells have inherent, built-in deficiencies, some of which compromise methyl metabolism, and this in turn leads to a gradual loss of DNA methylation. I proposed that these deficiencies and their effects are a mechanism of aging. As such, they would contribute to a finite cellular doubling potential, genetic instability, senescence, and cancer.

On the surface, having built-in inefficiencies in our DNA methylation system or in methyl metabolism seems like a cruel trick of nature. But if we look at it from an evolutionary point of view, it actually makes a lot of sense. Let's use mice as an example. In nature, most mice will either die of starvation or be killed by predators, disease, drought, or other environmental hazards long before they are greatly affected by aging. Likewise, those mice that survive to reproduce will generally do so well before they are greatly affected by aging. These considerations make a long-lived mouse unlikely and unnecessary. Why? Because it takes energy and crucial metabolites to keep an animal alive, and these would be better expended on immediate survival during the reproductive years of an animal's life. So in most animals all metabolism should be quite sufficient—in fact, optimized—for immediate and short-term needs such as youthful reproduction. This is a fundamental requirement of evolution. It should come as no surprise, then, that DNA methylation declines with age.

How does all this affect healthful longevity? The deficiencies in methyl metabolism probably exist from the time animals are young. A short-lived species such as the mouse would have evolved a more severe inherent deficiency in methyl metabolism than a long-lived species such as humans. Moreover—and this is important—these methylating deficiencies would have evolved in animals eating a balance of nutrients found in food from nature and would therefore be at least partially dependent on the diet. By manipulating the diet, especially in the direction of an increase in methylating nutrients, it may be possible to control these deficiencies.

When we're young we seem to have an excess of DNA

methylation, so that we can lose a significant amount before we begin to see adverse effects. This loss of DNA methylation would take many cell population doublings, because in each new generation of cells a relatively small fraction of methylation is lost. Think about a new car. It's got much more power than it needs simply to get you from one place to another. But as you drive it from year to year, it begins to lose some of that power. You don't really notice it, because the car can still get you to the grocery store. But eventually, if you don't take good care of it, your car stops running and won't get you anyplace at all. In the end, this reserve of methyl groups allows animals and cells to live long enough to reproduce and meet other evolutionary criteria. As long as those criteria are met, DNA methylation can decline, and both the animals and the cells they're made of can age.

There is good reason to think that this really happens. Some regions of DNA have high concentrations of sites where methylation can take place. These are often called *CG islands*. The number and length of CG islands tend to be greater in long-lived mammals such as humans than in short-lived mammals such as mice. Thus long-lived animals like humans have a greater potential to start out with a valuable "surplus" of methylation on some of these CG islands. That surplus could mean that it takes DNA methylation longer to run down and thus may help explain why some species live longer than others.

All these factors lead to the conclusion that better maintenance of DNA methylation will slow aging. In addition, eating a balance of nutrients shifted in favor of methyl metabolism should help maintain DNA methylation. If you want to accomplish this, it helps to eat a healthy diet as outlined in chapter 4. But diet alone—even a normal, balanced diet of foods from nature—won't supply enough methyl power to prevent declines in DNA methylation and thus slow aging and prevent or at least postpone age-related diseases.

To turn that trick, the best bet is to supplement your diet with folic acid, vitamin B_{12}, and betaine. This will help remethylate HCY and keep HCY in check. Meanwhile zinc assists the operation of three important enzymes in methylation, including the enzyme DNA methyltransferase that with SAM methylates our DNA. The *Methyl Magic* supplementation should produce higher SAM levels and SAM/SAH ratios than those found in a typical unsupplemented diet. Direct supplementation with SAM, though more expensive, should achieve the same result. The payoff is that *Methyl Magic* may well be the key to slowing down the process of aging and extending years of healthy life.

NUTRITION, HEALTH, AND LONGEVITY

We often hear it said—even by doctors and research scientists—that diet makes only a small difference in warding off the ravages of aging and extending life expectancy. These statements are often based on observations or studies of diets that can vary from country to country or even from individual to individual. But are any of these diets optimal for healthful longevity? *Definitely not!* At this point we don't really know what constitutes an optimal diet for healthful longevity, but we can be fairly certain that it bears little resemblance to the way most Americans eat now.

An optimal diet, which would include supplements or be made of engineered foods, would be designed to make sure we maintain our cells, organs, metabolism, and our health. While we don't yet know exactly what this optimal diet will look like, it will contain enough antioxidants to stop runaway oxidative damage early, while still allowing us to use oxidative processes that we need for energy, for defense against bacteria and viruses, and for signaling within and between cells. This optimal diet will have enough zinc, calcium, magnesium and other vital nutrients to keep the body's machinery running smoothly and to help keep us from losing bone mass as we age. Perhaps most important, this optimal diet will almost certainly keep HCY low and sustain methylation at reasonable levels. This in turn will presumably allow us to maintain our DNA methylation, our membrane fluidity, our protein repair, and a number of other vital functions that depend on methylation. The ultimate reward could well be lives extended toward or beyond our biologically allotted 100 to 120 years—*healthy* years, full of energy, achievement, and vitality.

We are all on a forced march. The route we travel is aging, and the road is full of pits and potholes, in the form of age-related killers like cancer and heart disease. We are only now beginning to understand the nature of these diseases and how we might slow them down. We can't expect to accomplish that with drugs alone. Nutrition, perhaps the most powerful of all medicines, will have to play a role. And the star players may very well turn out to be nutrients that boost methylation—folates, vitamins B_6 and B_{12}, betaine, choline, and the rest, the same nutrients that have been the focus throughout this book.

Is *Methyl Magic* the last word in living longer and slowing aging? Methylation is certainly one essential factor in slowing aging and living longer, but it is surely not the only means to that end. Once we develop an optimal diet, it's possible that humans could achieve life spans of as much as 150 years! Though we don't yet know all the details of an optimal diet, this book and others like it constitute a running start.

METHYL POWER SHOPPING TRIP

T he first stop on your *Methyl Magic* program should be your local supermarket or health food grocery. Here you'll find the foods that will lay the foundation for your program, a foundation on which you'll build with the special methyl-boosting supplements recommended in chapter 5. (The percentages quoted at the end of each entry are taken from actual foods as they are found in the supermarket. Foods can vary in their components, so these numbers are approximate.)

PRODUCE SECTION

This is where you should buy about one-half of your food. In other words, if you eat two thousand calories a day, about one thousand of them should come from fruits and vegetables. If you don't count calories, just take a look at your shopping cart on the way to the checkout stand. In this case *more* than half your bulk volume (of food) should come from the produce section.

RECOMMENDED PRODUCE

Most vegetables, including alfalfa sprouts, artichokes, asparagus, bamboo shoots, beans, beets, bok choy, broccoli, brussels sprouts, cabbage, carrots, cauliflower, celery, chervil, cilantro,

corn, cucumbers, dill, eggplant, escarole, garlic, ginger root, jicama, kale, leeks, lettuces, mushrooms, okra, onions, parsley,
peas, peppers, radicchio, radishes, seaweed, snow peas,
spinach, squash, string beans, sugar peas, sweet potatoes, Swiss
chard, turnips, water chestnuts, yams, and zucchini.

Vary these vegetables in your meals. Especially use
vegetables such as beans, cabbage, cauliflower, broccoli, bok
choy, brussels sprouts, kale, and spinach. These have plenty of
fiber, vitamins, and other essential nutrients. Note that white
or red potatoes are *not* on this recommended list, because of
their low fiber content. (Potatoes can still be okay in small
amounts—no more than 10 percent of your vegetable intake,
or one serving of potatoes for every twelve servings of other
vegetables.) Some of the vegetables listed here have about
half of carbohydrates as fiber (CAF1 about 50 percent, excellent) and less than 5 percent of calories as fat (CAF2 less than
5 percent, excellent).

Many fruits, including apples, apricots, bananas, blackberries,
blueberries, cantaloupe, cherries, dates, figs, grapes, mangoes,
melons, oranges, peaches, pears, pineapple, plums, prunes,
strawberries, and watermelon. These can be fresh and/or dried
fruits. Fruits are high in methyl-boosting nutrients like folic
acid, and they're also a great source of antioxidants. These
fruits generally have 10 to 25 percent of CAF1, with an average
of about 15 percent or higher (CAF1 about 15 percent, good).
Like the recommended vegetables, these fruits have less than
5 percent of calories as fat (CAF2 less than 5 percent, excellent).

In general all of these vegetables and fruits meet the
Methyl Magic dietary criteria, although vegetables should be
your top priority.

ACCEPTABLE PRODUCE

Avocados are mainly monounsaturated fat, which is
good, but they're also higher in calories than the vegetables in

the recommended list. Still, moderate amounts of avocado are good in the diet.

NOT RECOMMENDED PRODUCE

Potatoes or any other vegetable that is mainly starch with little fiber. Some corn products still have the germ and bran, which is good; however, others don't. Check the label for fiber content.

Note: As a small part of a meal that contains fiber from other sources (for example, potatoes in a dish with beans and broccoli, or as a "minority" vegetable in a vegetable soup), potatoes can be okay.

DRY FOODS AND CANNED FOODS SECTION

HIGHLY RECOMMENDED DRY AND CANNED FOODS

Beans and peas, including pinto beans, chickpeas, pink beans, white beans, black beans, navy beans, red beans, great northern beans, lima beans, lentils, garbanzo beans, black-eyed peas, red kidney beans, yellow split peas, and green split peas.

These beans and peas have a whopping 25 to 60 percent CAF1 (excellent), a good amount of protein, and little or no fat (CAF2 less than 5 percent, excellent). Beans also generally have lots of folate. Canning beans can reduce some of their vitamin content so starting with dry beans and cooking your own is most recommended. Beans have so much folate that even some loss from canning still leaves canned beans as a good source of folate.

Recommended bean products include canned kidney beans in salad, pork and beans (the amount of pork is usually very small), no-fat refried beans, soy flour (use in baking/cooking: for example, making pancakes, bread), bean soups, pea soups, hummus, and falafel.

A great thing about beans and bean products is that they can make a complete meal by themselves. They contain a good balance of protein, carbohydrate, and fiber. Beans, while excellent foods, actually have too little fat (except for soybeans), and while beans are high in protein, they don't have the best balance of amino acids for us (fish, poultry, and meat have a better amino acid balance). Therefore even though beans are an excellent food, use other foods (such as fish and green vegetables) a good part of the time. For maximum benefit, every time you eat a bean meal, make sure your next meal has some fish, poultry, dairy, egg, or meat.

Soups can have a complete and healthy balance of nutrients—especially soups with beans, peas, or lots of vegetables and some meat. Some examples:

- Split pea soup (for example, Campbell's Healthy Request Split Pea with Ham soup: ~23% protein by grams, ~14% CAF1, ~12% CAF2)
- Chicken vegetable soup (for example, Campbell's Chunky Hearty Chicken with Vegetable soup: ~30% protein by grams, ~17% CAF1, ~22% CAF2)

Chili: Most bean (no-meat) chilis are an excellent choice (check the label to be sure). Examples:

- Health Valley Vegetarian Chili (~32% protein by grams or calories, ~47% CAF1, no fat)
- Shelton's Turkey Chili with Beans (~39% protein by grams, 30% calories from protein, ~15% CAF1, ~15% CAF2)

RECOMMENDED DRY AND CANNED FOODS

Most canned produce is good, although fresh fruits and vegetables are even better. Check the label to make sure the manufacturer hasn't added a whole lot of salt and fat or sugar! Some vegetables, such as artichokes, bamboo shoots, beans, corn, peas, string beans, and water chestnuts, might be more available or more convenient in canned forms. Try to use mainly fresh produce with canned as a secondary source.

ACCEPTABLE DRY AND CANNED FOODS

Brown rice (about 10 percent CAF1, less than 5 percent CAF2) is acceptable, as are nuts and nut butters, including cashews, macadamia nuts, peanuts, almonds, and walnuts. Many of these nuts—including cashews, macadamia nuts, and peanuts—have healthy oils and can be used as a source of oils on some days (up to three days a week). Besides fat, another main component of nuts (generally) is protein. But take care: If you eat too many nuts, you'll get an excess of oil. If you are trying to lose or control your weight, treat nuts as an oil source (use in small amounts as recommended for oils) with a lower priority than fish, olive, or canola, oils.

NOT RECOMMENDED DRY AND CANNED FOODS

High sugar, corn syrup, or fat-added versions of canned fruits and vegetables. Check the label: either the section called "Nutrition Facts" or the ingredients list will tell you if the manufacturer has added sugars or fats.

Some examples of canned foods to avoid:

Fatty refried beans (20% CAF2), especially if that fat is lard or partially hydrogenated oils

Fatty bean dip with added partially hydrogenated oils: *read the label*

White rice has little fat (< 5% of total calories), but it also has very little fiber (< 3% of total carbohydrate). If you like white rice, it's okay in combination with vegetables, beans, or other high-fiber foods

Cream soups such as cream of chicken have up to 50 percent CAF2, in the forms of chicken fat, cow fat, and/or margarine; even cream of broccoli can have a ton of fat.

SPICES AND CONDIMENTS

Most spices are highly recommended. In fact, most spices are vegetables that just happen to be extremely flavorful. Many spices have antioxidants and a variety of healthy ingredients. In addition, spices are a healthy alternative to salt and fat for making food tasty.

Ketchups, mustards, relishes, and various sauces are usually A-okay. Unless you use huge amounts of them you will not significantly affect your diet. Usually the biggest downside to these foods is their salt and sugar content. Still, in small amounts with a meal you won't be getting enough of either to constitute a health hazard. Most of these products are fat-free, so they, like spices, provide a means of flavoring food without adding fat.

While we're at it, a note on salt (sodium chloride). Salt can be a hazard because it can cause an imbalance in your system between sodium and potassium, which in turn can contribute to high blood pressure. One way to avoid these hazards is to use Morton Lite salt, a mixture of sodium choride and potassium chloride. Another solution is to eat, and chew well, fresh vegetables and fruits—that way you'll get the potassium that's in their cells. Fruit and vegetable juices are also good sources of potassium. (By the way, you can't destroy potassium simply by heating it, but you can wash it away if you cook or blend foods and throw away their juices.)

OILS

Buy oils in small containers (that is, less than about 40 ounces), and store them in the refrigerator. Oils are liquid fat (in other words, 100 percent of their total calories are in the form of fat) and will have about 14 grams of fat per tablespoon. The key to keeping a lid on the saturated fat content is to pick the right oils. Any oil you plan to get very hot—especially by frying—should be high in monounsaturates, such as canola or olive.

(Some oils come with vitamin E added to preserve them, and that's good!)

RECOMMENDED OILS

Canola oil
Olive oil (a higher grade such as extra-virgin is probably best)
Soybean oil

ACCEPTABLE OILS

Peanut, macadamia nut oil, sesame, almond, avocado, safflower, and sunflower oils

NOT RECOMMENDED OILS

Corn oil, cottonseed oil, coconut, palm, beef fat, butter, lard (too high in artery-clogging saturated fats or have an imbalance among types of polyunsaturated fats)

SALAD DRESSINGS, MAYONNAISE, SALSAS, AND DIPS

RECOMMENDED SALAD DRESSINGS, MAYONNAISE, SALSAS, AND DIPS

Lots of salad dressings are now made with no fat or with soybean, olive, or canola oils, which contain heart-healthy monounsaturated and/or polyunsaturated fats. A tablespoon or less of these oils per day should be plenty. I prefer to make my own, so I know where the oil has been. Alternatively, shop at your health food store for a brand with a good reputation for quality, such as Spectrum or Hain.

Mayonnaise is similar. Use a fat-free or a soybean oil– or canola oil–based mayo. Again, a tablespoon or less per day should suffice.

Salsa contains about 30 percent of total CAF1. It's all vegetables (tomatoes and bell and jalapeño peppers) and no fat!

Hummus is also highly recommended, especially when made with olive, canola, or sesame oil. You can make your own hummus mix, with varying amounts of water and your own fresh olive oil (or canola or soybean). Or you can buy, for example, Fantastic Foods brand hummus mix (22 percent CAF1, 33 percent CAF2). Serve it with carrot sticks, zucchini, broccoli, cauliflower, bread, and crackers.

I also recommend bean dip, made either with no oil or with "healthy" canola or soybean oil.

ACCEPTABLE SALAD DRESSINGS, MAYONNAISE, SALSAS, AND DIPS

Yogurt-based dips or dips made with canola or soybean oils can be low in fat or made with healthy oils. (Remember, it's still possible to get too much "healthy" canola or soybean oil.) Don't exceed 30 percent of your total calories from fat, even if the fats come from these healthy oils. If you're exceptionally fond of dip, it's better to buy either the no-fat or very low-fat variety.

NOT RECOMMENDED SALAD DRESSINGS, MAYONNAISE, SALSAS, AND DIPS

Salad dressing with partially hydrogenated oil, cottonseed oil, or with much saturated fat

Mayonnaise with partially hydrogenated oil

Bean dip with added partially hydrogenated oil: read the
    label!

Sour cream–based dips

BREADS

Look for multigrain, whole-grain breads with at least
15 percent CAF1. I buy bread in the health food store; it's easier to find what I want there. I keep the ingredients list simple—nothing you need to have double majored in chemistry
and English to pronounce or understand. Enriched bread can
be okay; it has vitamins added, although it's usually made
with refined flour, which is lower in fiber. Store the bread in
the refrigerator (or long term in the freezer).

RECOMMENDED BREADS

Multigrain, whole-grain breads. One slice of these
breads might contain 4 grams of fiber, 20 grams carbohydrate, and 5 grams of protein. This means that about 20 percent of their carbohydrates are in the form of fiber (CAF1).
Also only about 5 percent of calories are in the form of fat
(CAF2). Try a five-grain bread, containing whole wheat, whole
barley, whole rye, whole oats, brown rice. Alternatively, look
for one-, two-, or ten-grain, whole-grain breads. (CAF1 and
CAF2 are similar to those just given for multigrain bread.)
Likewise aim for whole-grain hamburger buns, hot dog buns,
pita bread, or tortillas.

If you prefer white bread, try a more commercial
mixed refined and whole-grain bread with added fiber. Breads
with added fiber or made with soy flour can have plenty of
fiber even if they aren't whole grain. An example: Wonder
Light Wheat Bread. One slice has 6 grams of fiber and 18
grams of carbohydrate, so that CAF1 is about 33 percent and
CAF2 is about 6 percent. This is not typical white bread, so

check the label! Note also that "white" breads with added fiber and vitamins still don't have the preferred natural balance of fiber, vitamins, minerals, essential oils, et cetera, found in more complete whole-grain breads.

NOT RECOMMENDED BREADS

Avoid breads that are mainly "enriched" flour with little fiber and/or with added partially hydrogenated oils. This includes almost all "white" bread. For example, typical white bread contains less than 10 percent of total CAF1. Some white hamburger buns have only 4 percent of CAF1, and they contain added fat in the form of partially hydrogenated oil. Breadsticks are a little better (about 8 percent of CAF1), but they also have added fat. Packaged tube biscuits can have 10 percent of CAF1 but a whopping 40 percent of calories from fat. And supposedly healthy pita bread in its white form has only 3 percent of CAF1. These are examples—not all hamburger buns and the like have these same properties—so check the labels.

PASTA

RECOMMENDED PASTA

Whole-grain pastas with more than 15 percent CAF1. A good example: Hodgson Mill whole-wheat spirals.

ACCEPTABLE PASTA

Whole-grain pastas with more than 10 percent CAF1, such as Hodgson Mill whole-wheat noodles.

NOT RECOMMENDED PASTA

"Refined," "enriched" flour pasta or egg noodles with less than 10 percent CAF1.

CRACKERS

RECOMMENDED CRACKERS

Ak-mak brand whole-wheat crackers, 18 percent CAF1, 17 percent CAF2.

CONDITIONALLY ACCEPTABLE CRACKERS

Fat-free crackers: I find few crackers that really meet or come close to the basic criteria of more than 15 percent CAF1 and less than 30 percent CAF2, even in the health food store. However, crackers such as Nabisco Fat Free Premium Saltine Crackers—less than 10 percent CAF1, 0 percent CAF2 (no fat)—are okay *if* you eat them with a very fibrous meal—that is, with bean chili, split pea soup, or hummus dip. Again, as with bread, a whole-grain product is preferred.

NOT RECOMMENDED CRACKERS

Crackers with partially hydrogenated oils or those high in saturated fat.

SNACK FOODS

RECOMMENDED SNACK FOODS

Popcorn (24 percent CAF1): Just use a hot-air popper and then add your own canola or soybean oil (*not* hydrogenated) in a bowl after the corn is popped.

ACCEPTABLE SNACK FOODS

Baked Tostitos Tortilla Chips (8 percent CAF1, 5 percent CAF2): These don't have much fiber themselves, but if you have them with salsa and/or fat-free refried beans, you'll come out with flying colors!

BORDERLINE SNACK FOODS

Potato chips: These are actually a no-no because they have so little nutritional value. But if you must have them, you can find potato chips—especially in the health food store—made with canola oil (not hydrogenated) or high-oleic safflower oil. They still won't have much fiber. You will want to balance most chips with a low-fat, high-fiber carbohydrate source as well as some protein. The following chips are better than those in the Not Recommended category:

Reduced-fat potato chips by Ruffles (~ 5% CAF1, ~ 40% CAF2 as corn oil)

Chips cooked in canola oil or high-oleic safflower oil (these still have a lot of fat)

NOT RECOMMENDED SNACK FOODS

Pretzels ("enriched" flour), about 5 percent CAF1, 0 percent CAF2 (no fat); and chips with partially hydrogenated oil, cottonseed, palm, or coconut oils. Examples:

Potato chips (~5% CAF1, 50% CAF2 as partially hydrogenated oils): Don't confuse these with the acceptable chips in the previous section

Cheese puffs (~5% CAF1, 50% CAF2 as partially hydrogenated oils)

Corn chips (~5% CAF, 50% CAF2 as partially hydrogenated oils)

Tortilla chips (~5% CAF1, 50% CAF2 as partially hydrogenated oils)

Popular flavored tortilla chips (~5% CAF1, ~50% CAF2 as partially hydrogenated oils)

"Low-fat" potato chips with partially hydrogenated oils

Microwave popcorn: Looks okay until you get to the partially hydrogenated oils.

Beware the and/or oil list, as in "canola oil and/or partially hydrogenated cottonseed oil": Don't risk it!

PASTRIES AND COOKIES

RECOMMENDED PASTRIES AND COOKIES

Health Valley, Tree of Life, and Barbara's make a variety of cookies and other pastries that have plenty of fiber and are often fat-free, low in fat, or made with canola oil.

Look for whole-grain pastries and cookies that have more than 15 percent CAF1 and aim for canola oil and/or nuts as the fat source.

BORDERLINE PASTRIES AND COOKIES

Fat-free pastries and cookies. I find few pastries and cookies that have enough fiber, but if you do buy these products, at least pick a very low- or no-fat version. An example: fat-free breakfast tarts for the toaster (very little fiber but at least no fat).

NOT RECOMMENDED PASTRIES AND COOKIES

Pastries and cookies with little or no fiber and/or with partially hydrogenated oils and/or a lot of saturated fat. (Again, read the nutritional label and list of ingredients.) There are more of these than you can shake a stick of butter at (or, for that matter, than you can shake a sugar cane at). For example:

Snack cakes (no fiber and partially hydrogenated oil)

"Fitness" bars (< 10% CAF1)

Croissants (< 10% CAF1, 50% CAF2)

Breakfast tarts for the toaster (< 5% CAF1, 20–35% CAF2, including partially hydrogenated oil or cottonseed oil)

Low-fat breakfast tarts for the toaster (< 5% CAF1, 13% CAF2, including partially hydrogenated oil)

SEAFOOD

RECOMMENDED SEAFOOD

Most fresh, frozen, or canned fish, such as cod, tuna, orange roughy, swordfish, and salmon (but *not* breaded fish, which almost always has partially hydrogenated oil added. Even if they don't, breaded fish or meat will soak up extra oil when you fry them.) Tuna, cod, swordfish, and flounder may have less than 10 percent CAF2, and they're excellent protein sources. Other fish have more fat (salmon, for example, has 50 percent CAF2, but these are good monounsaturated and polyunsaturated fats).

Shrimp are basically all protein, with about 5 percent CAF2 (but *not* breaded shrimp).

ACCEPTABLE SEAFOOD

Sardines in tomato sauce (~ 40% CAF2, but these are mostly healthy monounsaturated fats from fish oil—sardines, tomato sauce, and chili pepper)

Imitation crab (15% CAF2, mostly carbohydrate)

Catfish (39% CAF2, but only about 7% calories as saturated fat)

MEATS

RECOMMENDED MEATS

No-fat or very low-fat meats. Note that it's an acceptable compromise to have some small amount of saturated fat in a protein-rich food like meat. Likewise it's an acceptable compromise to have low fiber with carbohydrate (low CAF1) in a protein-rich product with little or no fat.

By the way, check the prices on these and see if you don't get more protein for your money from the nonfat version than from the fat version. Why pay for saturated fat that you don't want anyway?

Tyson skinless chicken (25% CAF2)

Oven-roasted boneless breast of turkey (~ 10% CAF2)

Hickory-smoked breast of turkey (~ 17% CAF2)

Louis Rich Free—no-fat oven-roasted turkey breast slices (1 g carbohydrate per 4 g protein with no fat)

Oscar Mayer Free Hot Dogs (3 g carbohydrate per 6 g protein with no fat)

Soybeans and their products, which are often made into meat substitutes; they're healthy, and many taste good

Yves Veggie Pepperoni or Pizza Pepperoni or Veggie Wieners or Tofu Wieners (~70–80% protein, ~25–40% CAF1 and < 10% CAF2)

Boca Burgers (~57% protein, ~44% CAF1, ~9% CAF2)

Lightlife Gimme Lean! (~50% protein, ~12% CAF1, 0% CAF2)

Note: Bean products such as hummus or falafel or "veggie burgers" are good substitutes for meat on occasion.

ACCEPTABLE MEATS

Very lean beef, pork, lamb, chicken, turkey; for example:

"97% fat-free" turkey slices (33% CAF2)

Turkey breast (~35% CAF2)

NOT RECOMMENDED MEATS

Fatty cuts of any meat; for example:

Chicken breast with skin (~50% CAF2)

Chicken breast patties (~50% CAF2

Boneless strip steaks (60% CAF2)

Beef franks or hot dogs (~80% CAF2; I've even seen 90% CAF2 in some brands!)

Ham (~50% CAF2)

Premium ground turkey (50% CAF2)

Bacon (80% CAF2)

Pork sausage (80% CAF2)

Bologna (80% CAF2)

DAIRY

RECOMMENDED DAIRY PRODUCTS

No-fat or very low-fat dairy. Note that, as with meats, it's an acceptable compromise to have some small amount of saturated fat in a protein-rich food like dairy products. Likewise it's an acceptable compromise to have low fiber with carbohydrate (low CAF1) in a protein-rich product with little or no fat.

No-fat yogurt with moderate carbohydrate (that is, protein grams should be at least one-third of carbohydrate grams); a good example is Dannon Light

Low-fat yogurt (< 10% CAF2): Try Yoplait "99% fat free" yogurt

Skim milk (good protein and calcium source and 0% CAF2)

No-fat cottage cheese (or cottage cheese with < 10% CAF2)

Soy milk (available with various amounts of sugars, fat, and protein), e.g. EdenSoy

Fat-free cheese (examples: Healthy Choice Fat Free, Kraft Fat
Free)

ACCEPTABLE DAIRY PRODUCTS

Low-fat yogurt (< 20% CAF2)

"Low-fat" fat milk (~20% CAF2)

NOT RECOMMENDED DAIRY PRODUCTS

Butter: *All fat,* mostly (> 60%) saturated fat

Margarine: Usually all fat and/or partially hydrogenated oil

"2%" fat milk (maybe the manufacturers should call it 37% fat
milk, or 37% CAF2 milk!)

Whole milk (47% CAF2)

Cheese, mild cheddar (< 70% CAF2)

"Low-fat" cheese ("25% less fat than normal cheese," but
still > 50% CAF2)

Cream cheese (90% CAF2)

Cream

Sour cream (75% CAF2)

FROZEN FOODS SECTION

RECOMMENDED FROZEN FOODS

Frozen fish fillets (*not* breaded)

Frozen shrimp (*not* breaded)

ACCEPTABLE FROZEN FOODS

Various Healthy Choice brand products are low in fat
and have a reasonable amount of fiber.

BORDERLINE FROZEN FOODS

Some egg rolls, beef/rice/stir fry veggies, or beef and
bean burritos will have enough vegetables to be marginally acceptable.

NOT RECOMMENDED FROZEN FOODS

French fries (too little fiber, usually too much fat)

Pizza pepperoni and cheese: (< 10% CAF1, 40–50% CAF2)

Pastry-wrapped hot dogs on a stick or corndogs (< 10% CAF1, 50% CAF2)

Waffles (< 5% CAF1, 30% CAF2 using partially hydrogenated oil)

Chicken pot pies (< 10% CAF1, 60% CAF2)

Chili (some varieties contain 75% CAF2)

Sausage patties (> 80% CAF2!)

Biscuit, sausage, cheese, egg (< 10% CAF1, 60% CAF2)

Packaged meals: lunch packs with ham, cheese, crackers (< 5% CAF1, > 50% CAF2)

DELI

The deli section is like the rest of the supermarket, except without the labels. You're probably safest sticking with fish or skinless chicken and turkey products. Likewise hummus, bean salads, or sushi are probably some of your safer bets. For fiber pick something with lots of green veggies, beans, or peas.

BREAKFAST CEREALS

RECOMMENDED BREAKFAST CEREALS

Oatmeal, quick or slow versions (15% CAF1, 17% CAF2)

Shredded Wheat 'N Bran (17% CAF1, < 3% CAF2)

Raisin Bran (17% CAF1, 5% CAF2)

Oat bran hot cereal (25% CAF1, 20% CAF2)

Multigrain hot cereal (20% CAF1, 11% CAF2)

ACCEPTABLE BREAKFAST CEREALS:

Cheerios (13% CAF1, 14% CAF2)

Total (13% CAF1, < 10% CAF2)

Grape Nuts (11% CAF1, 5% CAF2)

NOT RECOMMENDED BREAKFAST CEREALS

Breakfast cereals with less than 5 percent CAF1 or with added fat are not recommended. Many breakfast cereals, by the way, are low in fat, but they are also often low in fiber.

I found one well-known example with less than 4 percent CAF1 (1 gram of fiber per 28 grams carbohydrate), added fat (as partially hydrogenated oil), and an ingredients list that looked like a chemical company catalog. This cereal actually had the symbol for meeting American Heart Association food criteria!

DESSERTS

RECOMMENDED DESSERTS

Fruits: strawberries, blueberries, cherries, apples, tangerines, and so on

Fruit cocktail in fruit juice (no added sugar)

High-fiber cookies, cakes, or pastries (such as those made by Tree of Life, Health Valley, or Barbara's)

ACCEPTABLE DESSERTS

Some of these have lots of sugar so make sure you have a balanced, fiberous meal first.

Rice Dream nondairy dessert such as cocoa marble fudge (~ 8% CAF1, 33% CAF2 as oleic safflower oil—a "good" oil)

Häagen-Dazs sorbet, no fat, almost no fiber or protein

Various fat-free ice creams: lots of carbohydrates, no fiber, but at least no fat

Fruit pie, pumpkin pie, and the like, if made with only moderate sugar and little or no fat

Note: Most pie crust is made with shortening or butter, so you will be getting some saturated fat.

NOT RECOMMENDED DESSERTS

Ice cream (0% CAF1, 50% CAF2—mostly saturated fat)

Cream pies (2% CAF1, 60% CAF2—mostly saturated and/or partially hydrogenated fat)

Most cakes (3% CAF1, 50% CAF2—mostly saturated and/or partially hydrogenated fat)

DRINKS

Drinks aren't expected to have much fiber, although some do. These drinks are rated based on their upsides (vitamins, minerals, protein) and downsides (sugar, saturated fat).

RECOMMENDED DRINKS

Just plain water, with or without ice

Mineral water (some types are a good mineral source, others just look nice)

Tea and coffee: Herbal tea and coffee have virtually no calories. Tea, especially green tea, has lots of beneficial antioxidants. If you're concerned about the caffeine content of coffee and some teas, keep in mind that caffeine increases blood circulation to the brain. On the other hand, if you have certain kinds of heart arrhythmias, anxiety, or panic disorders, you may want to avoid caffeine. And remember: "decaf" means "low caf," not "no caf."

Vegetable juices: tomato, V8 juice, and carrot juice; good examples are Campbell's tomato juice (~ 10% CAF1, no fat); V8 vegetable juice (~ 15% CAF1, no fat). *Some of these juices have more fiber than many bread or potato products!*

Soy milk (available with various amounts of sugars, fat, and protein), such as EdenSoy Organic Soy Beverage (27% CAF2 as soybean oil—lots of potassium, 31% calories from protein)

Skim milk—good protein and calcium source

Diet sodas (no benefit, but generally no great harm, either)

ACCEPTABLE DRINKS

Fruit juices have many beneficial ingredients. Orange juice, for example, has lots of folic acid, while grape juice contains significant amounts of choline. Fruit juices do have a great deal of sugar, which is why I dilute them until they're about half water.

Low-fat milk is a good source of protein and calcium, but it also has some saturated fat (about 20 percent CAF2)

NOT RECOMMENDED DRINKS:

"2% fat" milk: Good protein and calcium source (but contains ~37% CAF2, mainly saturated fat)

Whole milk: Good protein and calcium source (but contains ~47% CAF2, mainly saturated fat)

Regular sodas: (30–50 g of sugar per can and no fiber)

METHYL MAGIC RECIPES

H ere's a sample of some tasty *Methyl Magic* recipes: over fifteen items that will work for either lunch or dinner and a variety of breakfast suggestions. All of them will help you lay the dietary foundation for your *Methyl Magic* program, and some provide starter amounts of methyl-boosting ingredients. But remember, you can't get the full benefits of a *Methyl Magic* program through food alone. Along with these recipes—and others you may want to develop on your own—you'll want to take the dietary supplements listed in chapter 5.

Note: Some of these recipes use small amounts of potatoes, white crackers, and other low-fiber ingredients that are acceptable when they're used with high-fiber ingredients.

BREAKFAST

FRUIT AND YOGURT

Any fruit of choice: apples, apricots, bananas, blackberries, blueberries, cantaloupe, cherries, dates, figs, grapes, melons, oranges, peaches, pears, pineapple, plums, prunes, strawberries, or watermelon. These can be fresh and/or dried fruits.

Yogurt (low- or no-fat), preferably one higher in protein and lower in sugar. Look for a yogurt that contains 25 to 35 percent protein, with less than 20 percent CAF2.

CEREAL

Cold cereal: Shredded Wheat 'N Bran, Raisin Bran, Cheerios, Total, or Grape Nuts.

Hot cereal: oat bran or a multigrain, whole-grain, cereal.

Soy milk (such as EdenSoy) or skim cow's milk or low-fat cow's milk.

Serve with strawberries, blackberries, blueberries, cantaloupe, or other fruit.

This is light on the protein side. For more protein add *one* egg (prepared with no or moderate canola oil) or Lightlife Gimme Lean! brand meatless sausage (prepared with no or moderate canola oil).

BLUEBERRY PANCAKES

Ingredients

1 cup whole-grain wheat or buckwheat flour
1 cup cornmeal (whole-grain with germ and bran from either yellow or blue corn)
1 cup soy flour
2½ cups soy milk, soy-rice milk, or skim or low-fat cow's milk
3 eggs
1 cup blueberries (or chopped apples or chopped strawberries)
½ teaspoon Morton Lite salt
1½ tablespoons canola oil
4 teaspoons baking powder (*non*aluminum, such as Rumford's)
Canola oil for cooking

Directions

Mix ingredients to an even consistency in a bowl.

Add up to 1 cup of water if necessary to thin the batter. Cook on a griddle with a little canola oil.

This recipe has itself a fairly good balance of protein, carbohydrate, fiber, and fat. Makes eight to ten servings, eight to ten medium to large pancakes, enough for three to six individual meals. You may add moderate syrup (⅓ cup) or, for more protein, some Lightlife Gimme Lean! brand meatless sausage.

QUICK MEALS FOR LUNCH OR DINNER

SMOKY TOASTED FAST SANDWICH (LUNCH)

Ingredients
> 2 slices multigrain, whole-grain bread
> Sliced smoked ham or turkey (with < 30% CAF2)
> Head cabbage
> Wishbone Creamy Caesar dressing

Directions
> Toast the bread. Add two slices of meat to one slice of bread. Cut a ⅜-inch-thick (~1 cm) slice off the head of cabbage and place in the sandwich as if it were a big slice of tomato. Distribute about 1 tablespoon of dressing over this cabbage. Cover with second slice of bread, and enjoy.
> Makes two servings, enough for one meal.

TUNA SANDWICH (LUNCH)

Ingredients
> 6 ounces tuna in water
> ½ tablespoon mayonnaise (soy or canola oil–based)
> Pickles, finely diced (optional)
> Onion, finely diced (optional)
> 4 slices multigrain, whole-grain bread

Directions
> Mix tuna and mayo to an even consistency. Add diced pickle and/or onion, if desired. Spread on bread.

Serve with apple, carrots, sugar peas, and/or cauliflower.

Makes four servings, enough for two sandwiches. This sandwich has a fairly good balance of protein, carbohydrate, fiber, and fat. You may substitute leeks or garlic for onions. You may add a cabbage slice or kale leaves to the sandwiches for healthy variety.

VEGGIE BURGERS (LUNCH OR DINNER)

Ingredients

>Whole-wheat or multigrain hamburger buns
>Meatless "hamburgers" (such as Boca Burgers or
>>Lightlife Gimme Lean! brand meatless ground
>>"beef")
>Mustard, ketchup, lettuce, tomato, pickles

Directions

Microwave preformed and precooked patties or fry or grill ground meat substitute and assemble into "hamburgers."

HOT DOGS (DINNER OR LUNCH)

Ingredients

>Whole-wheat buns
>Hot dogs or soy dogs (for example, Yves Veggie or
>>Tofu Wieners or low-/no-fat meat hot dogs by
>>Healthy Choice, Oscar Mayer, or Hormel).
>Mustard, ketchup, relish

Directions

Microwave hot dogs and assemble.

BURRITO (DINNER OR LUNCH)

Ingredients

>Refried beans (low- or no-fat, such as Rosarita's No
>>Fat Zesty Salsa Refried Beans)
>Whole-wheat or corn tortillas

Sliced lettuce, tomatoes, mushrooms, and black
olives

Directions

Place refried beans on tortilla and microwave. Add
lettuce, tomatoes, mushrooms, black olives, and wrap
up. Serve with salsa or guacamole (smooshed avocados
mixed with salsa).

FISH OR CHICKEN WITH SALAD
OR STEAMED VEGGIES (DINNER OR LUNCH)

Grill or broil fish or chicken (4 to 6 ounces). Place on
¼ to ⅓ of a standard (about 10-inch-diameter) dinner
plate. Cover the rest of the plate with a large mixed green
salad and/or with mixed lightly steamed vegetables. Use
one of the salad dressings offered in this recipe section, or
use a tablespoon or less of a prepared dressing made with
canola, olive, or soybean oil.

Fruit (about 1 cup) for dessert.

LUNCH OR DINNER CHOICES

ORLEANS-MADRAS HOT FISH (DINNER OR LUNCH)

Ingredients

1 tablespoon canola oil

2 teaspoons curry powder

16 ounces fish (cod, pollack, roughy, or other white
ocean fish, fresh or frozen)

½ medium white or red onion, sliced

2 teaspoons Cajun spice mix (such as Paul Prud-
homme's Blackened Redfish Magic)

Directions

In a frying pan heat the oil at medium to medium-
high heat, then add the curry powder and sauté until it
just starts to darken (roughly 20 seconds, depending on

heat). Quickly distribute oil and curry in the pan and add fish. Distribute onions around fish. Let fish and onions cook until fish is about half-done. Sprinkle Cajun spice on the fish, then turn the fish over and sprinkle with Cajun spice again. Cook until fish is done.

Serve with a large mixed green salad and fruit. (Salad dressing recipes are at the end of this section.) Makes six to eight servings, enough for two to four individual meals.

LITTLE ROCK CATFISH (DINNER OR LUNCH)

Ingredients

> 16 ounces fish (catfish, cod, pollack, or roughy, fresh or frozen)
> 1 tablespoon olive oil
> ½ cup each of
>> Chopped broccoli
>> Diced onions (white, yellow, or red)
>> Sliced green bell peppers
>> Raisins
>> Sliced mushrooms
>> Chopped cabbage
> 1 apple (Golden, Red Delicious, or Fuji), sliced
> 6 green olives (without pits)
> 1 cup pasta sauce (such as Classico Mushrooms and Ripe Olives)

Directions

Grill, broil, or fry fish. In a frying pan, heat the oil at medium to medium-high heat. Sauté the broccoli, onions, peppers, raisins, mushrooms, cabbage, and apple. Add the fish, green olives, and pasta sauce. Stir, cover, and simmer for 10 minutes on low heat.

Serve with green salad.

Makes 6 to 8 servings, enough for two to four individual meals. You may substitute chicken for fish in this recipe.

FISH AND VEGETABLE CURRY (DINNER OR LUNCH)

Ingredients

- 2 teaspoons olive oil
- 2 teaspoons canola oil
- 2 teaspoons curry powder
- ⅛ teaspoon Chinese angelica root powder (optional)
- 16 ounces fish (cod, pollack, roughy, or other white ocean fish, fresh or frozen)
- ½ medium yellow onion, diced
- ½ medium red onion, diced
- ⅓ head cabbage, sliced
- 2 medium yellow squash, sliced lengthwise
- 5 medium mushrooms, diced
- 2 Fuji apples, sliced

Directions

In a frying pan, heat the oil at medium to medium-high heat. Once heated, add the curry powder and sauté until it *just starts* to darken (roughly 20 seconds, depending on heat). Quickly add angelica root (optional). Distribute oil in the pan and add fish. Distribute onions around fish. Let fish and onions cook about 2 minutes, then add the cabbage, squash, mushrooms, and apples. With pan 75 percent covered, let fry on medium heat for another few minutes (until fish is about half-done). Turn over fish and flip or stir the rest. Let cook with pan 90 percent covered for another several minutes until fish is done.

Serve with grapes, peaches, yams, or sweet potatoes.

Makes six to eight servings, enough for two to four individual meals. You may substitute chicken for fish in this recipe.

QUICK SPICY FISH (DINNER OR LUNCH)

Ingredients

- 1 tablespoon canola oil
- 16 ounces orange roughy or other white ocean fish

½ cup white or red onion, diced
¼ teaspoon powdered ginger
Dash of red pepper
3 cups chopped broccoli crowns
24 ounces pasta sauce (such as Classico Tomato and
  Basil)

Directions

In a frying pan, heat the oil at medium to medium-high heat. Once heated, add fish and onions and let cook until fish is about half-done. Sprinkle ginger and red pepper on the fish. Turn the fish over and sprinkle ginger and red pepper again. Add broccoli, cover pan about 80 percent, and lower heat slightly.

Cook until fish is done (broccoli should be lightly steamed at this point). Break up fish with a spatula, add pasta sauce, and mix. Heat until sauce is warm.

Makes four to six servings, enough for two to three individual meals.

KIM'S CHILI (DINNER OR LUNCH)

Ingredients

Three varieties of canned beans (14- to 17-ounce can
  of each):
  black beans
  baked beans
  pinto beans or pork and beans
½ onion, diced
4 garlic cloves, diced
⅓ cup cumin
1 can Rotel diced tomatoes and green chilies
1 tomato, diced
1 tablespoon fresh chopped or dried basil

Directions

Combine all ingredients. Simmer 15 to 20 minutes.

In place of canned beans you can start with a total of

16 ounces of dry beans and soak for at least one hour ahead of time. Using 1 teaspoon of baking soda in the soak can improve the cooking rate for dry beans. Use soak solution for the chili—it will have the vitamins you want.

Have this with salad or vegetables (or by itself, since Kim's Chili is a balanced meal). For healthy oils you can mix in canola, olive, or soybean oil (preferably after chili is cooked). For more protein add some fat-free shredded cheese. For more zing you can top with chopped onions. For crackers use Ak-mak brand. However, there's enough fiber in Kim's Chili that you can have Nabisco Fat Free Premium Saltine Crackers if you want to use "white bread" crackers.

Makes eight to ten servings, enough for three to five individual meals.

MULLIGATAWNY STEW (DINNER OR LUNCH)

Ingredients
- 1 teaspoon powdered ginger root
- 1 teaspoon garam masala (ground spice mix of coriander, cumin, ginger, cloves, black pepper, cardamom, cinnamon, pimento, bay leaves, and nutmeg)
- ½ teaspoon coriander powder
- ½ teaspoon cumin powder
- ½ teaspoon red chili powder
- ½ teaspoon turmeric powder
- 1 tablespoon canola oil
- 1 medium red onion, diced
- 1 medium white onion, diced
- 1 medium apple (Golden Delicious or Fuji), chopped
- 1 small white or red potato, chopped
- 2 cups dry yellow lentils (soak in water for 3 or more hours before cooking or used canned)

2 cups dry chick peas (soak in water for 3 or more
hours before cooking or use canned)
1 quart chicken broth
½ leek, thinly sliced
2 medium cloves garlic
1 tablespoon soy sauce
2 tablespoons Lea & Perrins Worcestershire Sauce

Directions

Sauté spices (ginger, garam masala, coriander, cumin, chili, and tumeric) briefly in the canola oil on medium heat, then add onions, apple, and potato, mix and sauté briefly, then cover and leave on low to medium heat to steam for about 5 minutes. Add everything to a large pot with a cover and heat. Bring just to a boil and then simmer for 3 or more hours. When soaking dry peas or lentils, 1 or 2 teaspoons of baking soda in the soak can improve the cooking rate. Use the soak solution for the stew—it will have the vitamins you want.

Serve with fruit such as peaches, mangoes, melon, or grapes, and with crackers or pita bread.

Makes ten to twelve servings, enough for four to six individual meals.

PASTA WITH "ALFREDO" SAUCE (DINNER OR UNCH)

"Alfredo" Sauce Ingredients

1½ tablespoons olive oil
1½ tablespoons mayonnaise (soy or canola
oil–based)
3 tablespoons white vinegar (can substitute lemon
juice)
1 tablespoon sesame tahini
2 tablespoons soy milk (such as EdenSoy) or skim
cow's milk

Additional Ingredients
- 8 ounces fish or chicken
- 1 cup chopped cauliflower or other preferred vegetable
- ¼ cup fresh basil or cilantro
- ½ teaspoon olive oil
- ¼ teaspoon Morton Lite salt
- 10 ounces whole-grain pasta or pasta with soy flour added (for example, Hodgson Mill whole-wheat noodles or spirals or Contadina white durum flour and soy flour linguine)

"Alfredo" Sauce Directions

Combine and mix all ingredients to even consistency.

Additional Directions

Grill, broil, or fry fish or chicken. Steam or grill cauliflower or other vegetable. Boil pot of water and add ½ teaspoon olive oil and ¼ teaspoon Morton Lite salt. Add pasta to boiling water, cook until done, and drain pasta. Add sauce, fish or chicken, and vegetable.

Serve with fresh basil or cilantro. You can add a little Parmesan cheese if you prefer. Also, variations can include other vegetables, such as artichokes, broccoli, garlic, onions, yellow squash, and zucchini.

Makes four to six servings, enough for portions of two to four individual meals.

PASTA WITH TOMATO SAUCE (DINNER OR LUNCH)

Ingredients
- 8 ounces fish, chicken, or soy-based meat substitute (for example, Lightlife Gimme Lean! brand meatless sausage)
- ½ teaspoon olive oil
- ¼ teaspoon Morton Lite salt

10 ounces whole-grain pasta or pasta with soy flour
   added (for example, Hodgson Mill whole-wheat
   noodles or spirals or Contadina white durum
   flour and soy flour linguine)
24 ounces pasta sauce (for example, Classico Tomato
   and Basil or Mushrooms and Ripe Olives)
¾ cup chopped broccoli or other preferred vegetable
Sprig of fresh cilantro or basil (optional)

Directions

Grill, broil, or fry fish, chicken, or soy-based meat substitute. Boil pot of water and add olive oil and Morton Lite salt. Add pasta, cook until done, and drain. Add sauce and broccoli. Heat until warm/hot.

Serve with fresh cilantro or basil. You can add a little Parmesan cheese if you prefer. Also, variations can include other vegetables such as artichokes, cauliflower, garlic, onions, yellow squash, and zucchini.

Makes six to eight servings, enough for portions of two to four individual meals

PIZZA (DINNER OR LUNCH)

Ingredients for Dough

1½ cups warm water
1 tablespoon active dry yeast
1 teaspoon honey
1⅓ cups unbleached white wheat flour
1⅓ cups soy flour
1⅓ cups whole-wheat flour
½ teaspoon salt
Pinch of basil
Pinch of parsley

Ingredients for Topping

1 cup canned or fresh tomato sauce (for example,
   Classico Tomato and Basil Pasta Sauce)

½ red onion, sliced
1 teaspoon thyme, dried or fresh, chopped
2 teaspoons chopped fresh basil
1 teaspoon chopped fresh parsley
1 teaspoon oregano, dried or fresh, chopped
1 teaspoon minced fresh garlic
1 teaspoon black pepper
¼ teaspoon salt
Pinch of sugar
1 cup sliced mushrooms
⅓ zucchini, sliced ⅛-inch thick
⅓ yellow squash, sliced ⅛-inch thick
½ cup broccoli
1 tomato, sliced ⅛-inch thick (vine ripened or organic)
1 cup shredded low-fat cheese (for example, Healthy
    Choice Mozzarella cheese, 30% CAF2)
Ives Pizza Pepperoni (soy based)
2 ounces anchovies (optional)

Directions

In a large bowl, combine the water, yeast, and honey. In a separate bowl, combine the flours. Add 4 teaspoons of the flour mixture to the water, yeast and honey mixture. Stir gently. Cover the bowl with a damp towel and let stand for 30 minutes in a warm place. This mixture should become foamy.

Add a pinch of basil, a pinch of parsley, the salt, and the rest of the flour. Knead for around 10 minutes until the dough is well combined. Add a bit of additional flour should the dough become sticky. Place the dough in a large bowl. Cover this with a damp towel in a warm place for about 45 minutes. Punch the dough down and roll to fit a 16-inch pizza pan.

Preheat the oven to 400 degrees. In a large bowl, combine tomato sauce, onions, thyme, basil, parsley, oregano, garlic, pepper, salt, and sugar. Spread this mixture over the dough on the pizza pan.

Layer the cheese, zucchini, yellow squash, broccoli, tomato, mushrooms, pepperoni, anchovies (optional), and any additional toppings over the sauce. Bake the pizza for 15 to 20 minutes until crust is brown.

Top pizza with your favorite vegetables, such as peppers and olives. The dough can be frozen for up to two months. The sauce can be kept refrigerated for up to three days. Makes one 16-inch pizza; serves four to six.

OCEANSIDE TACOS (DINNER OR LUNCH)

Ingredients

    16 ounces fish (cod, pollack, roughy, or swordfish, fresh or frozen)

    ⅛ head of cabbage, sliced

    ½ onion, diced

    1 large or 2 small tomatoes, diced

    4 tablespoons fresh, chopped cilantro

    Whole-wheat tortilla or corn tortilla shells

Directions

Grill, broil, or fry fish. Assemble as you would any taco, adding the fish, cabbage, onion, tomato, and cilantro. (You may substitute chicken or falafels for fish in this recipe or substitute pita bread for tortillas.) Add White Sauce for fish, chicken, or falafels (see following recipe) or salsa (such as Pace Medium).

Makes six to eight servings, enough for two to four individual meals.

WHITE SAUCE (FOR FISH, CHICKEN, OR FALAFELS)

Ingredients

    3 tablespoons mayonnaise (soy or canola oil–based)

    3 tablespoons white vinegar (can substitute lemon juice)

1 tablespoon sesame tahini

2 tablespoons soy milk (e.g. EdenSoy) or skim cow's
milk

Directions

Combine and mix all ingredients to even consistency. Have this with fish or chicken, as in Oceanside Tacos.

About half the volume of White Sauce consists of healthy oils (canola, soybean, and sesame oil). Two tablespoons of White Sauce will supply an adequate amount of healthy oils for one day. For flavor variations, add ¼ teaspoon of either Worcestershire sauce, molasses, sesame oil, or finely ground white pepper.

MISO SOUP (LUNCH OR DINNER)

Ingredients

3 or 4 shiitake mushrooms (fresh or dried)

1 gram hijiki seaweed

3 ounces firm tofu

1 medium spring (green) onion, finely chopped

1 tablespoon miso (traditional red Japanese fermented soy product)

1 quart water (for the soup)

2 cups water to soak mushrooms

⅓ cup water to dissolve miso

Morton Lite salt (to taste)

Directions

Soak shiitake mushrooms for 20 minutes in about 2 cups of water, then discard the soaking water and the stems, and slice the mushrooms. Soak hijiki seaweed for 20 minutes in the 1 quart of water for the soup. Dice the tofu into small cubes about ¼ inch on each side. Combine the mushrooms, tofu, and onion with the seaweed in water, bring to a boil, then simmer for 20 minutes to make "stock." Just before serving, mix and dissolve the miso in about ⅓ cup of water and add 1 or 2 tablespoons of this dissolved miso to each bowl for individual servings of soup. You may add Morton Lite salt to taste (¼ teaspoon per quart of soup). Then ladle into each individual serving bowl 1 to 2 cups of the hot mushrooms, tofu, onion, and seaweed "stock." Serve immediately.

Makes about six individual servings of soup. Have with sushi, sandwich, or other main course.

CABBAGE SALAD (DINNER OR LUNCH)

Ingredients

⅓ head red cabbage, sliced

⅓ head green cabbage, sliced

5 medium mushrooms, sliced

¼ red onion, diced

1 tablespoon olive oil

1 teaspoon sesame oil

1 tablespoon Nakano seasoned rice vinegar

Dash of white pepper

Sprig of fresh cilantro or basil (optional)

Directions

Combine ingredients, mix, and serve with fish, chicken, kidney beans or other protein source for a complete dinner or lunch. Note: Variations can include other vegetables, such as artichokes, bok choy, broccoli, cauliflower, cucumbers, jicama, parsley, and zucchini.

Makes about six servings, enough for portions of two to four individual meals.

SESAME SALAD DRESSING

Ingredients

1 tablespoon olive oil

1 teaspoon sesame oil

1 tablespoon Nakano seasoned rice vinegar

Dash of white pepper

Directions

Combine ingredients and mix well before pouring on salad.

Makes one or two servings, depending on your healthy oil needs.

BASIL RED PEPPER SALAD DRESSING

Ingredients

1 tablespoon apple cider vinegar

1 tablespoon olive oil

1 teaspoon Miracle Whip

¼ teaspoon basil (fresh or dry)

Dash of red pepper

Directions

Combine ingredients and mix well before pouring on salad. Makes one or two servings, depending on your healthy oil needs.

You can vary the type and amount of oil in these dressing recipes to suit your taste and needs.

SNACKS

HUMMUS DIP

Ingredients

¾ cup hummus mix (for example, Fantastic Foods brand)

¼ cup olive oil

¼ cup white vinegar

½ cup water

1 teaspoon chopped garlic (fresh or dried), optional

1 teaspoon chopped basil (fresh or dried), optional

1 teaspoon chopped cilantro (fresh or dried), optional

Directions

Mix to an even consistency. You can make this mix with variable amounts of water, vinegar, and oil to adjust to your preferred consistency or to adjust CAF2. You can add some sesame oil for flavor or use canola or soybean oil. For better flavor when using dried spices, leave the finished hummus in the refrigerator for 1 hour to overnight to let the spices rehydrate.

Serve with carrot sticks, zucchini, broccoli, cauliflower, bread, and/or crackers, or stuff into mushrooms.

REFRIED BEAN DIP AND SALSA

Microwave no-fat refried beans (for example, Rosarita's No Fat Zesty Salsa Refried Beans). Top with no-fat shredded cheese (optional). Serve with salsa (for example, Pace brand) and baked tortilla chips (for example, Frito-Lay Baked Tostitos).

MISCELLANEOUS

Keep a few of these around to snack on: pickles, peppers, apples, bananas, figs, prunes, dried mixed fruits, zucchini, carrots, string peas/beans, snow peas, mushrooms, celery, cauliflower, broccoli, chewing gum, diet soda, tea, mineral water, vegetable juices, and diluted fruit juice.

METHYL RESOURCES

A variety of information on new clinical tests and other new developments in methylation, health, and longevity are available on the Methyl Magic Web site:

www.methylmagic.com

This site also has important links to other methylation, health, and longevity resources.

Research on methylation and longevity holds enormous promise to enrich, strengthen, and lengthen our lives. There is a nonprofit foundation just for this purpose. If you would like to help methylation and longevity research, please send your contribution to the Methylation Research Institute Foundation at the following address:

Methylation Research Institute
P.O. Box 123
Little Rock, AR 72203

Please make checks payable to the MRI Foundation.

The Foundation also has a Web site:
www.methyl.org

The SAM test, as well as other tests discussed in *Methyl Magic,* are available from Specialty Laboratories. Specialty offers nearly 4,000 different assays for the assessment and monitoring of patient health. For more information on the SAM test and related assays, please have your physician contact Specialty Laboratories' client services at 1-800-421-7110 and on the Web at www.specialtylabs.com.

Betaine (TMG), SAM, and other nutritional supplements in a wide and innovative variety are available from Life Extension Foundation. Life Extension also provides a variety of clinical testing and information on health and longevity. You can reach Life Extension at 1-800-544-4440 and on the Web at www.lef.org.

REFERENCES

CHAPTER 2

Blusztajn, J. K. 1998. Choline, a vital amine. *Science* 281, 794–95.

Boelsterli, U. A., Rakhit, G., Balazs, T. 1983. Modulation by S-adenosyl-L-methionine of hepatic Na+,K+-ATPase, membrane fluidity, and bile flow in rats with ethinyl estradiol-induced cholestasis. *Hepatology* 3, 12–17.

Cimino, M., Vantini, G., Algeri, S., Curatola, G., Pezzoli, C., Stramentinoli, G. 1984. Age-related modification of dopaminergic and beta-Adrenergic receptor system: restoration to normal activity by modifying membrane fluidity with S-adenosylmethionine. *Life Sci* 34, 2,029–39.

Haworth, J. C., Dilling, L. A., Surtees, R. A., Seargeant, L. E., Lue-Shing, H., Cooper, B. A., Rosenblatt, D. S. 1993. Symptomatic and asymptomatic methylenetetrahydrofolate reductase deficiency in two adult brothers. *Am J Med Genet* 45, 572–76.

Hirata, F., Axelrod, J. 1980. Phospholipid methylation and biological signal transmission. *Science* 209, 1,082–90.

Kim, S., Lim, I. K., Park, G. H., Paik, W. K. 1997. Biological methylation of myelin basic protein: enzymology and biological significance. *Int J Biochem Cell Biol* 29, 743–51.

LeBlanc, M. J., Gavino, V., Perea, A., Yousef, I. M., Levy, E., Tuchweber, B. 1998. The role of dietary choline in the beneficial effects of lecithin on the secretion of biliary lipids in rats. *Biochim Biophys Acta* 1393, 223–34.

Okinaga, S., Ohrui, T., Nakazawa, H., Yamauchi, K., Sakurai, E., Watanabe, T., Sekizawa, K., Sasaki, H. 1995. The role of HMT (histamine N-methyltransferase) in airways: a review. *Methods Find Exp Clin Pharmacol* 17 (suppl. C), 16–20.

Pyeritz, R. E. 1993. Homocystinuria. In Beighton P. (ed.), *McKusick's Heritable Disorders of Connective Tissue* (St. Louis, C.V. Mosby), 137–78.

Refsum, H., Ueland, P. M., Nygard, O., Vollset, S. E. 1998. Homocysteine and cardiovascular disease. *Annu Rev Med* 49, 31–62.

Sitaram, B. R., Sitaram, M., Traut, M., Chapman, C. B. 1995. Nyctohemeral rhythm in the levels of S-adenosylmethionine in the rat pineal gland and its relationship to melatonin biosynthesis. *J Neurochem* 65 1,887–94.

Thompson, P. A., Shields, P. G., Freudenheim, J. L., Stone, A., Vena, J. E., Marshall, J. R., Graham, S., Laughlin, R., Nemoto, T., Kadlubar, F. F., Ambrosone, C. B. 1998. Genetic polymorphisms in catechol-O-methyltransferase, menopausal status, and breast cancer risk. *Cancer Res* 58, 2,107–10.

CHAPTER 3

Bostom, A. G., Roubenoff, R., Dellaripa, P., Nadeau, M. R., Sutherland, P., Wilson, P. W., Jacques, P. F., Selhub, J., Rosenberg, I. H. 1995. Validation of abbreviated oral methionine-loading test. *Clin Chem,* 41, 948–49.

Brouwer, D. A., Welten, H. T., Reijngoud, D. J., van Doormaal, J. J., Muskiet, F. A. 1998. Plasma folic acid cutoff value, derived from its relationship with homocyst(e)ine. *Clin Chem* 44, 1,545–50.

Cooney, C. A., Wise, C. W., Poirier, L. A. 1997. An improved sample preparation method for the quantitative HPLC determination of 5-methyldeoxycytidine in animal tissue DNA. *J Liq Chrom* 20, 1,279–93.

Loehrer, F. M., Schwab, R., Angst, C. P., Haefeli. W. E., Fowler, B. 1997. Influence of oral S-adenosylmethionine on plasma 5-methyltetrahydrofolate, S-adenosylhomocysteine, homocysteine and methionine in healthy humans. *J Pharmacol Exp Ther* 282, 845–50.

Silberberg, J., Crooks, R., Fryer, J., Wlodarczyk, J., Nair, B., Guo, X. W., Xie, L. J., Dudman, N. 1997. Gender differences and other determinants of the rise in plasma homocysteine after L-methionine loading. *Atherosclerosis* 133, 105–10.

Van der Griend, R., Haas, F. J., Duran, M., Biesma, D. H., Meuwissen, O. J., Banga, J. D. 1998. Methionine-loading test is necessary for detection of hyperhomocysteinemia. *J Lab Clin Med* 132, 67–72.

Wise, C. K., Cooney, C. A., Ali, S. F., Poirier, L. A. 1997. Measuring S-adenosylmethionine in whole blood, red blood cells and cultured cells using a fast preparation method and high-performance liquid chromatography. *J Chromatogr B Biomed Sci Appl* 696, 145–52.

CHAPTER 4

Ascherio, A., Willett, W. C. 1997. Health effects of trans-fatty acids. *American Journal of Clinical Nutrition* 66, 1,006S–10S.

Giovannucci, E., Stampfer, M. J., Colditz, G. A., Rimm, E. B., Trichopoulos, D., Rosner, B. A., Speizer, F. E., Willett, W. C. 1993. Folate, methionine, and alcohol intake and risk of colorectal adenoma. *J Natl Canc Inst* 85, 875–84.

Hu, F. B., Stampfer, M. J., Manson, J. E., Rimm, E., Colditz, G. A., Rosner, B. A., Hennekens, C. H., Willett, W. C. 1997. Dietary fat intake and the risk of coronary heart disease in women. *New England Journal of Medicine* 337, 1,491–99.

Millian, N. S., Garrow, T. A. 1998. Human betaine-homocysteine methyltransferase is a zinc metalloenzyme. *Arch Biochem Biophys* 356, 93–98.

Orentreich, N., Matias, J. R., DeFelice, A., Zimmerman, J. A. 1993. Low methionine ingestion by rats extends life span. *Journal of Nutrition* 123, 269–74.

Reeves, P. G., Nielsen, F. H., Fahey, G. C. Jr. 1993. AIN-93 purified diets for laboratory rodents: final report of the American Institute of Nutrition ad hoc writing committee on the reformulation of the AIN-76A rodent diet. *Journal of Nutrition* 123, 1,939–51.

Rimm, E. B., Willett, W. C., Hu, F. B., Sampson, L., Colditz, G. A., Manson, J. E., Hennekens, C., Stampfer, M. J. 1998. Folate and vitamin B_6 from diet and supplements in relation to risk of coronary heart disease among women. *JAMA* 279, 359–64.

Simopoulos, A. P. 1997. Omega-3 fatty acids in the prevention-management of cardiovascular disease. *Canadian Journal Physiology and Pharmacology* 75, 234–39.

Zeisel, S. H., and Blusztajn, J. K. 1994. Choline and Human Nutrition. *Annual Review of Nutrition* 14, 269–96.

CHAPTER 5

Bernstein, A. L. 1990. Vitamin B_6 in clinical neurology. *Ann N Y Acad Sci* 585, 250–60.

Bestor, T. H. 1992. Activation of mammalian DNA methyltransferase by cleavage of a Zn binding regulatory domain. *EMBO J* 11 2,611–17.

Christen, S., Woodall, A. A., Shigenaga, M. K., Southwell-Keely, P. T., Duncan, M. W., Ames, B. N. 1997. Gamma-tocopherol traps mutagenic electrophiles such as NO(X) and complements alpha-tocopherol: physiological implications. *Proc Natl Acad Sci USA* 94, 3,217–22.

Clarke, R., Frost, C., Leroy, V., Collins, R. Lowering blood homocysteine with folic acid based supplements: meta-analysis of randomised trials. *BMJ* 316, 894–98.

Cooney, C. A. 1993. Are somatic cells inherently deficient in methylation metabolism? A proposed mechanism for DNA methylation loss, senescence and aging. *Growth, Dev & Aging* 57, 261–73.

Duell, P. B., Malinow, M. R. 1997. Homocyst(e)ine: an important risk factor for atherosclerotic vascular disease.*Curr Opin Lipidol* 8, 28–34.

Holme, E., Kjellman, B., Ronge, E. 1989. Betaine for treatment of homocystinuria caused by methylenetetrahydrofolate reductase deficiency. *Arch Dis Child* 64, 1,061–64.

Kuzminski, A. M., Del Giacco, E. J., Allen, R. H., Stabler, S. P., Lindenbaum, J. 1998. Effective treatment of cobalamin deficiency with oral cobalamin. *Blood* 92, 1,191–98.

Meydani, M., Meisler, J. G. 1997. A closer look at vitamin E. Can this antioxidant prevent chronic diseases? *Postgrad Med* 102, 199–201.

Refsum, H., Ueland, P. M., Nygard, O., Vollset, S. E. 1998. Homocysteine and cardiovascular disease. *Annu Rev Med* 49, 31–62.

Storch, K. J., Wagner, D. A., Young, V. R. 1991. Methionine kinetics in adult men: effects of dietary betaine on L-[2H3-methyl-1-13C]methionine. *American Journal of Clinical Nutrition* 54, 386–94.

Wendel, U., Bremer, H. J. 1984. Betaine in the treatment of homocystinuria due to 5,10-methylenetetrahydrofolate reductase deficiency. *Eur J Pediatr* 142, 147–50.

Zeisel, S. H., Blusztajn, J. K. 1994. Choline and human nutrition. *Annual Review of Nutrition* 14, 269–96.

CHAPTER 6

Conlay, L. A., Sabounjian, L. A., Wurtman, R. J. 1992. Exercise and neuromodulators: choline and acetylcholine in marathon runners. *Intl. J. Sports Med.* 13, S141–42.

Conlay, L. A., Wurtman, R. J., Blusztajn, K., Coviella, I. L., Maher, T. J., Evoniuk, G. E. 1986. Decreased plasma choline concentrations in marathon runners. *N Engl J Med* 315, 892.

Nygoard, O., Vollset, S. E., Refsum, H., Stensvold, I., Tverdal, A., Nordrehaug, J. E., Ueland, P. M., Kvoale, G. 1995. Total plasma homocysteine and cardiovascular risk profile the Hordaland Homocysteine Study Journal of the American Medical Association *JAMA* 274, 1,526–33.

Toler, S. M. 1997. Creatine is an ergogen for anaerobic exercise. *Nutrition Reviews* 55, 21.

CHAPTER 7

Barak, A. J., Beckenhauer, H. C., Tuma, D. J. 1996. Betaine, ethanol, and the liver: a review. *Alcohol* 13, 395–98.

Cravo, M. L., Gloria, L. M., Selhub, J., Nadeau, M. R., Camilo, M. E., Resende, M. P., Cardoso, J. N., Leitao, C. N., Mira, F. C. 1996. Hyperhomocysteinemia in chronic alcoholism: correlation with folate, vitamin B_{12}, and vitamin B_6 status. *Am J Clin Nutr* 63, 220–24.

Giovannucci, E., Stampfer, M. J., Colditz, G. A., Rimm, E. B., Trichopoulos, D., Rosner, B. A., Speizer, F. E., Willett, W. C. 1993. Folate, methionine, and alcohol intake and risk of colorectal adenoma. *J Natl Canc Inst* 85, 875–84.

Hultberg, B., Berglund, M., Andersson, A., Frank, A. 1993. Elevated plasma homocysteine in alcoholics. *Alcohol Clin Exp Res* 17, 687–89.

Rimm, E. B., Willett, W. C., Hu, F. B., Sampson, L., Colditz, G. A., Manson, J. E., Hennekens, C., Stampfer, M. J. 1998. Folate and vitamin B_6 from diet and supplements in relation to risk of coronary heart disease among women. *JAMA* 279, 359–64.

CHAPTER 8

Blusztajn, J. K. 1998. Choline, a vital amine. *Science* 281, 794–95.

Brush, M. G., Bennett, T., Hansen, K. 1988. Pyridoxine in the treatment of premenstrual syndrome: a retrospective survey in 630 patients. *Br J Clin Pract* 42, 448–52.

Butterworth, C. E. Jr., Hatch, K. D., Macaluso, M., Cole, P., Sauberlich, H. E., Soong, S. J., Borst, M., Baker, V. V. 1992. Folate deficiency and cervical dysplasia. *JAMA*, 267, 528–33.

Cermak, J. M., Holler, T., Jackson, D. A., Blusztajn, J. K. 1998. Prenatal availability of choline modifies development of the hippocampal cholinergic system. *FASEB J* 12, 349–57.

Confavreux, C., Hutchinson, M., Hours, M. M., Cortinovis-Tourniaire, P., Moreau, T. 1998. Rate of pregnancy-related relapse in multiple sclerosis: pregnancy in multiple sclerosis group. *N Engl J Med* 339, 285–91.

Dekker, G. A., de Vries, J. I., Doelitzsch, P. M., Huijgens, P. C., von Blomberg, B. M., Jakobs, C., van Geijn, H. P. 1995. Underlying disorders associated with severe early-onset preeclampsia. *Am J Obstet Gynecol* 173, 1,042–48.

Doll, H., Brown, S., Thurston, A., Vessey, M. 1989. Pyridoxine (vitamin B_6) and the premenstrual syndrome: a randomized crossover trial. *J R Coll Gen Pract* 39, 364–68.

Eskes, T. K. 1998. Neural tube defects, vitamins and homocysteine. *Eur J Pediatr* 157 Suppl 2, S139–41.

Frezza, M., Centini, G., Cammareri, G., Le Grazie, C., Di Padova, C. 1990. S-adenosylmethionine for the treatment of intrahepatic cholestasis of pregnancy. Results of a controlled clinical trial. *Hepatogastroenterology* 37 (suppl. 2), 122–25.

Garner, S. C., Mar, M. H., Zeisel, S. H. 1995. Choline distribution and metabolism in pregnant rats and fetuses are influenced by the choline content of the maternal diet. *J Nutr* 125, 2,851–58.

Jacob, R. A., Gretz, D. M., Taylor, P. C., James, S. J., Pogribny, I. P., Miller, B. J., Henning, S. M., Swendseid, M. E. 1998. Moderate folate depletion increases plasma homocysteine and decreases lymphocyte DNA methylation in postmenopausal women. *J Nutr* 128, 1,204–12.

Liu, T., Soong, S. J., Wilson, N. P., Craig, C. B., Cole, P., Macaluso, M., Butterworth, C. E. 1993. A case control study of nutritional factors and cervical dysplasia. *Cancer Epidemiol Biomarkers Prev* 2, 525–30.

Manzi, S., Meilahn, E. N., Rairie, J. E., Conte, C. G., Medsger, T. A. Jr., Jansen-McWilliams, L., D'Agostino, R. B., Kuller, L. H. 1997. Age-specific incidence rates of myocardial infarction and angina in women with systemic lupus erythematosus: comparison with the Framingham Study. *Am J Epidemiol* 145, 408–15.

McCarty, D. J., Manzi, S., Medsger, T. A. Jr., Ramsey-Goldman, R., LaPorte, R. E., Kwoh, C. K. 1995. Incidence of systemic lupus erythematosus. Race and gender differences. *Arthritis Rheum* 38, 1,260–70.

Meck, W. H., Smith, R. A., Williams, C. L. 1989. Organizational changes in cholinergic activity and enhanced visuospatial memory as a function of choline administered prenatally or postnatally or both. *Behav Neurosci* 103, 1,234–41.

Mijatovic, V., Kenemans, P., Jakobs, C., van Baal, W. M., Peters-Muller, E. R., van der Mooren, M. J. 1998. A randomized controlled study of the effects of 17beta-estradiol-dydrogesterone on plasma homocysteine in postmenopausal women. *Obstet Gynecol* 91, 432–36.

Molloy, A. M., Mills, J. L., Kirke, P. N., Ramsbottom, D., McPartlin, J. M., Burke, H., Conley, M., Whitehead, A. S., Weir, D. G., Scott, J. M. 1998. Low blood folates in NTD pregnancies are only partly explained by thermolabile 5,10-methylenetetrahydrofolate reductase: low folate status alone may be the critical factor. *Am J Med Genet* 78, 155–59.

Nygard, O., Refsum, H., Ueland, P. M., Vollset, S. E. 1998. Major lifestyle determinants of plasma total homocysteine distribution: the Hordaland Homocysteine Study. *Am J Clin Nutr* 67, 263–70.

Rimm, E. B., Willett, W. C., Hu, F. B., Sampson, L., Colditz, G. A., Manson, J. E., Hennekens, C., Stampfer, M. J. 1998. Folate and vitamin B_6 from diet and supplements in relation to risk of coronary heart disease among women. *JAMA* 279, 359–64.

Steegers-Theunissen, R. P., Boers, G. H., Steegers, E. A., Trijbels, F. J., Thomas, C. M., Eskes, T. K. 1992. Effects of sub-50 oral contraceptives on homocysteine metabolism: a preliminary study. *Contraception* 45, 129–39.

Steen, M. T., Boddie, A. M., Fisher, A. J., Macmahon, M., Saxe, D., Sullivan, K. M., Dembure, P. P., Elsas, L. J. 1998. Neural-tube defects are associated with low concentrations of cobalamin (vitamin B_{12}) in amniotic fluid. *Prenat Diagn* 18, 545–55.

Williams, C. L., Meck, W. H., Heyer, D. D., Loy, R. 1998. Hypertrophy of basal forebrain neurons and enhanced visuospatial memory in perinatally choline-supplemented rats. *Brain Res* 794, 225–38.

Yung, R., Powers, D., Johnson, K., Amento, E., Carr, D., Laing, T., Yang, J., Chang, S., Hemati, N., Richardson, B. 1996. Mechanisms of drug-induced lupus. II. T-cells overexpressing lymphocyte function-associated antigen 1 become autoreactive and cause a lupuslike disease in syngeneic mice. *J Clin Invest* 97, 2,866–71.

Zeisel, S. H., Mar, M. H., Zhou, Z., da Costa, K. A. 1995. Pregnancy and lactation are associated with diminished concentrations of choline and its metabolites in rat liver. *J Nutr.* 125, 3,049–54.

CHAPTER 9

Bestor, T. H. 1998. The host defence function of genomic methylation patterns. *Novartis Found Symp* 214, 187–95.

Cimino, M., Vantini, G., Algeri, S., Curatola, G., Pezzoli, C., Stramentinoli, G. 1984. Age-related modification of dopaminergic and beta-Adrenergic receptor system: restoration to normal activity by modifying membrane fluidity with S-adenosylme-thionine. *Life Sci* 34, 2,029–39.

Hirata, F., Axelrod, J. 1980. Phospholipid methylation and biological signal transmission. *Science* 209, 1,082–90.

Kim, E., Lowenson, J. D., MacLaren, D. C., Clarke, S., Young, S. G. 1997. Deficiency of a protein-repair enzyme results in the accumulation of altered proteins, retardation of growth, and fatal seizures in mice. *Proc Natl Acad Sci USA* 94, 6,132–37.

Kim, S., Lim, I. K., Park, G. H., Paik, W. K. 1997. Biological methylation of myelin basic protein: enzymology and biological significance. *Int J Biochem Cell Biol* 29, 743–51.

Li, E., Bestor, T. H., Jaenisch, R. 1992. Targeted mutation of the DNA methyltransferase gene results in embryonic lethality. *Cell* 69, 915–26.

Pyeritz, R. E. 1993. Homocystinuria. In Beighton P. (ed.), *McKusick's Heritable Disorders of Connective Tissue* (St. Louis, C. V. Mosby), 137–78.

Tate, P., Skarnes, W., Bird, A. 1996. The methyl-CpG binding protein MeCP2 is essential for embryonic development in the mouse. *Nat Genet* 12, 205–8.

Wolff, G. L., Kodell, R. L., Moore, S. R., Cooney, C. A. 1998. Maternal epigenetics and methyl supplements affect *agouti* gene expression in A^{vy}/a Mice. *FASEB J* 12, 949–57.

CHAPTER 10

Boushey, C. J., Beresford, S. A. A., Omenn, G. S., Motulsky, A. G. 1995. Quantitative assessment of plasma homocysteine as a risk factor for vascular disease: probable benefits of increasing folic acid intakes. *Journal of the American Medical Association* 274, 1,049–57.

Duell, P. B., Malinow, M. R. 1997. Homocyst(e)ine: an important risk factor for atherosclerotic vascular disease. *Curr Opin Lipidol* 8, 28–34.

McCully, K. S. 1992. Homocystinuria, arteriosclerosis, methylmalonic aciduria, and methyltransferase deficiency: a key case revisited. *Nutr Rev* 50, 7–12.

McCully, K. S. 1997. *The Homocysteine Revolution* (Keats Publishing).

Morrison, H. I., Schaubel, D., Desmeules, M., Wigle, D. T. 1996. Serum folate and risk of fatal coronary heart disease. *JAMA* 275, 1,893–96.

Munshi, M. N., Stone, A., Fink, L., Fonseca, V. 1996. Hyperhomocysteinemia following a methionine load in patients with non-insulin-dependent diabetes mellitus and macrovascular disease. *Metabolism* 45, 133–35.

Nygoard, O., Vollset, S. E., Refsum, H., Stensvold, I., Tverdal, A., Nordrehaug, J. E., Ueland, P. M., Kvoale, G. 1995. Total plasma homocysteine and cardiovascular risk profile the Hordaland Homocysteine Study Journal of the American Medical Association *JAMA* 274, 1,526–33.

Refsum, H., Ueland, P. M., Nygard, O., Vollset, S. E. 1998. Homocysteine and cardiovascular disease. *Annu Rev Med* 49 31–62.

Perry, I. J., Refsum, H., Morris, R. W., Ebrahim, S. B., Ueland, P. M., Shaper, A. G. 1995. Prospective study of serum total homocysteine concentration and risk of stroke in middle-aged British men. *Lancet* 346, 1,395–98.

Selhub, J., Jacques, P. F., Bostom, A. G., D'Agostino, R. B., Wilson, P. W., Belanger, A. J., O'Leary, D. H., Wolf, P. A., Schaefer, E. J., Rosenberg, I. H. 1995. Association between plasma homocysteine concentrations and extracranial carotid-artery stenosis. *N Engl J Med* 332, 286–91.

Southern, F. N., Cruz, N., Fink, L. M., Cooney, C. A., Barone, G. W., Eidt, J. F., Moursi, M. M. 1998. Hyperhomocysteinemia increases intimal hyperplasia in a rat carotid endarterectomy model. *J Vasc Surg 28,* 909–18.

Stampfer, M. J., Malinow, M. R., Willett, W. C., Newcomer, L. M., Upson, B., Ullman, D., Tishler, P. V., Hennekens, C. H. 1992. A prospective study of plasma homocyst(e)ine and risk of myocardial infarction in US physicians. *JAMA* 268, 877–81.

Tsai, J. C., Perrella, M. A., Yoshizumi, M., Hsieh, C. M., Haber, E., Schlegel, R., Lee, M. E. 1994. Promotion of vascular smooth muscle cell growth by homocysteine: a link to atherosclerosis. *Proc Natl Acad Sci USA* 91, 6,369–73.

Wang, H., Yoshizumi, M., Lai, K., Tsai, J. C., Perrella, M. A., Haber, E., Lee, M. E. 1997. Inhibition of growth and p21ras methylation in vascular endothelial cells by homocysteine but not cysteine. *J Biol Chem* 272, 25,380–85.

Wilgram, G. F., Hartroft, W. S., Best, C. H. 1954. Abnormal lipid in coronary arteries and aortic sclerosis in young rats fed a choline-deficient diet. *Science* 119, 842–43.

CHAPTER 11

Baylin, S. B., Herman, J. G., Graff, J. R., Vertino, P. M., Issa, J. P. 1998. Alterations in DNA methylation: a fundamental aspect of neoplasia. *Adv Cancer Res* 72, 141–96.

Blount, B. C., Mack, M. M., Wehr, C. M., MacGregor, J. T., Hiatt, R. A., Wang, G., Wickramasinghe, S. N., Everson, R. B., Ames, B. N. 1997. Folate deficiency causes uracil misincorporation into human DNA and chromosome breakage: implications for cancer and neuronal damage. *Proc Natl Acad Sci USA* 94, 3,290–95.

Branda, R. F., Nigels, E., Lafayette, A. R., Hacker, M. 1998. Nutritional folate status influences the efficacy and toxicity of chemotherapy in rats. *Blood* 92, 2,471–76.

Cooney, C. A. 1993. Are somatic cells inherently deficient in methylation metabolism? A proposed mechanism for DNA methylation loss, senescence and aging. *Growth, Dev & Aging 57*, 261–73.

Counts, J. L., Sarmiento, J. I., Harbison, M. L., Downing, J. C., McClain, R. M., Goodman, J. L. 1996. Cell proliferation and global methylation status changes in mouse liver after phenobarbital and/or choline-devoid, methionine-deficient diet administration. *Carcinogenesis* 17, 1,251–57.

Counts, J. L., Goodman, J. I. 1995. Hypomethylation of DNA: a possible epigenetic mechanism involved in tumor promotion. *Prog Clin Biol Res* 391, 81–101.

Fenech, M. F., Dreosti, I. E., Rinaldi, J. R. 1997. Folate, vitamin B_{12}, homocysteine status and chromosome damage rate in lymphocytes of older men. *Carcinogenesis* 18, 1,329–36.

Fenech, M., Aitken, C., Rinaldi, J. 1998. Folate, vitamin B_{12}, homocysteine status and DNA damage in young Australian adults. *Carcinogenesis* 19, 1,163–71.

Gama-Sosa, M. A., Slagel, V. A., Trewyn, R. W., Oxenhandler, R., Kuo, K. C., Gehrke, C. W., Ehrlich, M. 1983. The 5-methylcytosine content of DNA from human tumors. *Nucleic Acids Res* 11, 6,883–94.

Giovannucci, E., Stampfer, M. J., Colditz, G. A., Rimm, E. B., Trichopoulos, D., Rosner, B. A., Speizer, F. E., Willett, W. C. 1993. Folate, methionine, and alcohol intake and risk of colorectal adenoma. *J Natl Canc Inst* 85, 875–84.

Giovannucci, E., Stampfer, M. J., Colditz, G. A., Hunter, D. J., Fuchs, C., Rosner, B. A., Speizer, F. E., Willett, W. C. 1998. Multivitamin use, folate, and colon cancer in women in the Nurses Health Study. *Ann Intern Med* 129, 517–24.

Jacob, R. A., Gretz, D. M., Taylor, P. C., James, S. J., Pogribny, I. P., Miller, B. J., Henning, S. M., Swendseid, M. E. 1998. Moderate folate depletion increases plasma homocysteine and decreases lymphocyte DNA methylation in postmenopausal women. *J Nutr* 128, 1,204–12.

Pascale, R. M., Marras, V., Simile, M. M., Daino, L., Pinna, G., Bennati, S., Carta, M., Seddaiu, M. A., Massarelli, G., Feo, F. 1992. Chemoprevention of rat liver carcinogenesis by S-adenosyl-L-methionine: A long-term study. *Canc Res* 52, 4,979–86.

Pascale, R. M., Simile, M. M., De Miglio, M. R., Nufris, A., Daino, L., Seddaiu, M. A., Rao, P. M., Rajalakshmi, S., Sarma, D. S., Feo, F. 1995. Chemoprevention by S-adenosyl-L-methionine of rat liver carcinogenesis initiated by 1,2-dimethylhydrazine and promoted by orotic acid. *Carcinogenesis* 16, 427–30.

Pogribny, I. P., Basnakian, A. G., Miller, B. J., Lopatina, N. G., Poirier, L. A., James, S. J. 1995. Breaks in genomic DNA and within the p53 gene are associated with hypomethylation in livers of folate/methyl-deficient rats. *Cancer Res* 55, 1,894–1,901.

Poirier, L. A. 1994. Methyl group deficiency in hepatocarcinogenesis. *Drug Metabolism Reviews* 26, 185–99.

Romanov, G. A., Vanyushin, B. F. 1981. Methylation of reiterated sequences in mammalian DNAs. Effects of the tissue type, age, malignancy and hormonal induction. *Biochim Biophys Acta* 653, 204–18.

Shin, O. H., Mar, M. H., Albright, C. D., Citarella, M. T., da Costa, K. A., Zeisel, S. H. 1997. Methyl-group donors cannot prevent apoptotic death of rat hepatocytes induced by choline-deficiency. *J Cell Biochem* 64, 196–208.

Simile, M. M., Saviozzi, M., De Miglio, M. R., Muroni, M. R., Nufris, A., Pascale, R. M., Malvaldi, G., Feo, F. 1996. Persistent chemopreventive effect of S-adenosyl-L-methionine on the development of liver putative preneoplastic lesions induced by thiobenzamide in diethylnitrosamine-initiated rats. *Carcinogenesis* 17, 1,533–37.

Wilson, M. J., Shivapurkar, N., Poirier, L. A. 1984. Hypomethylation of hepatic nuclear DNA in rats fed with a carcinogenic methyl-deficient diet. *Biochem J* 218, 987–90.

CHAPTER 12

Di Padova, C. 1987. S-adenosylmethionine in the treatment of osteoarthritis: review of the clinical studies. *Am J Med* 83 (suppl. 5A), 60–65.

Gutierrez, S., Palacios, I., Sánchez-Pernaute, O., Hernández, P., Moreno, J., Egido, J., Herrero-Beaumont, G. 1997. SAMe restores the changes in the proliferation and in the synthesis of fibronectin and proteoglycans induced by tumour necrosis factor alpha on cultured rabbit synovial cells. *Br J Rheumatol*, 36, 27–31.

Kim, Y. I., Logan, J. W., Mason, J. B., Roubenoff, R. 1996. DNA hypomethylation in inflammatory arthritis: reversal with methotrexate. *J Lab Clin Med* 128:2, 165–72.

Stone, J., Doube, A., Dudson, D., Wallace, J. 1997. Inadequate calcium, folic acid, vitamin E, zinc, and selenium intake in rheumatoid arthritis patients: results of a dietary survey. *Semin Arthritis Rheum* 27, 180–85.

Yung, R. L., Johnson, K. J., Richardson, B. C. 1995. New concepts in the pathogenesis of drug-induced lupus. *Lab Invest* 73, 746–59.

Yung, R. L., Quddus, J., Chrisp, C. E., Johnson, K. J., Richardson, B. C. 1995. Mechanism of drug-induced lupus. I. Cloned Th2 cells modified with DNA methylation inhibitors in vitro cause autoimmunity in vivo. *J Immunol* 154, 3,025–35.

CHAPTER 13

Bottiglieri, T., Hyland, D., Reynolds, E. H. 1994. The clinical potential of ademetionine (S-adenosylmethionine) in neurological disorders. *Drugs* 48, 137–52.

Esparza, M. L., Sasaki, S., Kesteloot, H. 1995. Nutrition, latitude, and multiple sclerosis mortality: an ecologic study. *Am J Epidemiol* 142, 733–37.

Frequin, S. T., Wevers, R. A., Braam, M., Barkhof, F., Hommes, O. R. 1993. Decreased vitamin B_{12} and folate levels in cerebrospinal fluid and serum of multiple sclerosis patients after high-dose intravenous methylprednisolone. *J Neurol* 240, 305.

Jacobson, W., Saich, T., Borysiewicz, L. K., Behan, W. M., Behan, P. O., Wreghitt, T. G. 1993. Serum folate and chronic fatigue syndrome. *Neurology* 43, 2,645–47.

Müller, F., Svardal, A. M., Aukrust, P., Berge, R. K., Ueland, P. M., Froland, S. S. 1996. Elevated plasma concentration of reduced homocysteine in patients with human immunodeficiency virus infection. *Am J Clin Nutr* 63, 242–48.

Nijst, T. Q., Wevers, R. A., Schoonderwaldt, H. C., Hommes, O. R., de Haan, A. F. 1990. Vitamin B_{12} and folate concentrations in serum and cerebrospinal fluid of neurological patients with special reference to multiple sclerosis and dementia. *J Neurol Neurosurg Psychiatry* 53, 951–54.

Reynolds, E. H. 1992. Multiple sclerosis and vitamin B_{12} metabolism. *J Neuroimmunol* 40, 225–30.

Schilling, R. F., Williams, W. J. 1995. Vitamin B_{12} deficiency: under-diagnosed, overtreated? *Hosp Pract* (off ed) 30, 47–52.

Surtees, R. 1998. Demyelination and inborn errors of the single carbon transfer pathway. *Eur J Pediatr* 157 Suppl 2, S118– 21.

Tang, A. M., Graham, N. M., Chandra, R. K., Saah, A. J. 1997. Low serum vitamin B_{12} concentrations are associated with faster human immunodeficiency virus type 1 (HIV-1) disease progression. *J Nutr* 127, 345–51.

Tavoni, A., Vitali, C., Bombardieri, S., Pasero, G. 1987. Evaluation of S-adenosylmethionine in primary fibromyalgia. A double-blind crossover study. *Am J Med* 83, 107–10.

CHAPTER 14

Alpert, J. E., Fava, M. 1997. Nutrition and depression: the role of folate. *Nutr Rev* 55, 145–49.

Bottiglieri, T. 1996. Folate, vitamin B_{12} and neuropsychiatric disorders. *Nutrition Reviews* 54, 382–90.

Bressa, G. M. 1994. S-adenosyl-l-methionine (SAMe) as antidepressant: meta-analysis of clinical studies. *Acta Neurol Scand Suppl* 154, 7–14.

Cohen, S. M., Nichols, A., Wyatt, R., Pollin, W. 1974. The administration of methionine to chronic schizophrenic patients: a review of ten studies. *Biol Psychiatry* 8, 209–25.

Drachman, D. A., Leavitt, J. 1994. Human memory and the cholinergic system. *Arch Neurol* 30, 113–21.

Fava, M., Borus, J. S., Alpert, J. E., Nierenberg, A. A., Rosenbaum, J. F., Bottiglieri, T. 1997. Folate, vitamin B_{12}, and homocysteine in major depressive disorder. *Am J Psychiatry* 154, 426–28.

Freeman, J. M., Finkelstein, J. D., Mudd, S. H. 1975. Folate-responsive homocystinuria and "schizophrenia.": a defect in methylation due to deficient 5,10-methylenetetrahydrofolate reductase activity. *N Engl J Med* 292, 491–96.

Godfrey, P. S., Toone, B. K., Carney, M. W., Flynn, T. G., Bottiglieri, T., Laundy, M., Chanarin, I., Reynolds, E. H. 1990. Enhancement of recovery from psychiatric illness by methylfolate. *Lancet* 336, 392–95.

Hasanah, C. I., Khan, U. A., Musalmah, M., Razali, S., M. 1997. Reduced red-cell folate in mania. *J Affect Disord* 46, 95–99.

Kagan, B. L., Sultzer, D. L., Rosenlicht, N., Gerner, R. H. 1990. Oral S-adenosylmethionine in depression: a randomized, double-blind, placebo-controlled trial. *Am J Psychiatry* 147, 591–95.

Lindenbaum, J., Healton, E. B., Savage, D. G., Brust, J. C., Garrett, T. J., Podell, E. R., Marcell, P. D., Stabler, S. P., Allen, R. H. 1988. Neuropsychiatric disorders caused by cobalamin deficiency in the absence of anemia or macrocytosis. *N Engl J Med* 318, 1,720–28.

Meck, W., Church, R. 1987. Nutrients that modify the speed of internal clock and memory storage processes. *Behav Neuroscience* 101, 465–75.

Ravakhah, K., West, B. C. 1995. Case report: subacute combined degeneration of the spinal cord from folate deficiency. *Am J Med Sci* 310, 214–16.

Regland, B., Johansson, B. V., Gottfries, C. G. 1994. Homocysteinemia and schizophrenia as a case of methylation deficiency. *J Neural Transm Gen Sect* 98, 143–52.

Sitaram, N., Weingartner, H., Gillin, J. C. 1978. Human serial learning: enhancement with arecholine and choline impairment with scopolamine. *Science* 201, 274–76.

Sitaram, N., Weingartner, H., Caine, E. D., Gillin, J. C. 1978. Choline: selective enhancement of serial learning and encoding of low imagery words in man. *Life Sci* 22 1,555–60.

Solama, R., Prudo-Alcala, R. A. 1990. Retrograde amnesia produced by intrastriatal atropine and its reversal by choline. *Lif Sci* 46, 679–86.

Spillman, M., Fava, M. 1996. S-adenosylmethionine (ademetionine) in psychiatric disorders. *CNS Drugs* 6, 416–25.

Susser, E., Brown, A. S., Klonowski, E., Allen, R. H., Lindenbaum, J. 1998. Schizophrenia and impaired homocysteine metabolism: a possible association. *Biol Psychiatry* 44, 141–43.

Wecker, L. 1988. Influence of dietary choline availability and neuronal demand on acetylcholine synthesis by rat brain. *J Neurochem* 51, 497–504.

Wecker, L. 1986 Neurochemical effects of choline supplementation. *Can J Physiol Pharmacol* 64:3, 329–33.

Williams, C. L., Meck, W. H., Heyer, D. D., Loy, R. 1998. Hypertrophy of basal forebrain neurons and enhanced visuospatial memory in perinatally choline-supplemented rats. *Brain Res* 794, 225–38.

CHAPTER 15

Allen, R. H., Stabler, S. P., Lindenbaum, J. 1998. Relevance of vitamins, homocysteine and other metabolites in neuropsychiatric disorders. *Eur J Pediatr* 157 (suppl. 2), S122–26.

Blusztajn, J. K. 1998. Choline, a vital amine. *Science* 281, 794–95.

Blusztajn, J. K., Holbrook, P. G., Lakher, M., Liscovitch, M., Maire, J. C., Mauron, C., Richardson, U. I., Tacconi, M., Wurtman, R. J. 1986. "Autocannibalism" of membrane choline-phospholipids: physiology and pathology. *Psychopharmacol Bull* 22, 781–86.

Brattstrom, L., Lindgren, A., Israelsson, B., Andersson, A., Hultberg, B. 1994. Homocysteine and cysteine: determinants of plasma levels in middle-aged and elderly subjects. *J Intern Med* 236, 633–41.

Cohen, B. M., Renshaw, P. F., Stoll, A. L., Wurtman, R. J., Yurgelun-Todd, D., Babb, S. M. 1995. Decreased brain choline uptake in older adults: an in vivo proton magnetic resonance spectroscopy study. *JAMA* 274, 902–7.

Cooney, C. A. 1993. Are somatic cells inherently deficient in methylation metabolism? A proposed mechanism for DNA methylation loss, senescence and aging. *Growth, Dev & Aging* 57, 261–73.

Cooney, C. A. 1994. Methylation metabolism has a central role in mammalian longevity. *AGE* 17, 166–67.

Finch, C. E. 1990. *Longevity, Senescence and the Genome* (Chicago: University of Chicago Press).

Holliday, R. 1986. Strong effects of 5-azacytidine on the in vitro life-span of human diploid fibroblasts. *Exp Cell Res* 166, 543–52.

Kodama, T., Mizobuchi, M., Takeda, R., Torikai, H., Shinomiya, H., Ohashi, Y. 1995. Hampered expression of isoaspartyl protein carboxyl methyltransferase gene in the human cataractous lens. *Biochim Biophys Acta* 1,245, 269–72.

Mijatovic, V., Kenemans, P., Jakobs, C., van Baal, W. M., Peters-Muller, E. R., van der Mooren, M. J. 1998. A randomized controlled study of the effects of 17beta-estradiol-dydrogesterone on plasma homocysteine in postmenopausal women. *Obstet Gynecol* 91, 432–36.

Ortega, R. M., Mañas, L. R., Andrés, P., Gaspar, M. J., Agudo, F. R., Jiménez, A., Pascual, T. 1996. Functional and psychic deterioration in elderly people may be aggravated by folate deficiency. *J Nutr* 126, 1,992–99.

Riggs, K. M., Spiro, A. III, Tucker, K., Rush, D. 1996. Relations of vitamin B_{12}, vitamin B_6, folate, and homocysteine to cognitive performance in the Normative Aging Study. *Am J Clin Nutr* 63, 306–14.

Singhal, R. P., Mays-Hoopes, L. L., Eichhorn, G. L. 1987. DNA methylation in aging of mice. *Mech Ageing Dev* 41, 199–210.

Ulus, I. H., Wurtman, R. J., Mauron, C., Blusztajn, J. K. 1989. Choline increases acetylcholine release and protects against the stimulation-induced decrease in phosphatide levels within membranes of rat corpus striatum. *Brain Res* 484, 217–27.

Vanyushin, B. F., Nemirovsky, L. E., Klimenko, V. V., Vasiliev, V. K., Belozersky, A. N. 1973. The 5-methylcytosine in DNA of rats: tissue and age specificity and the changes induced by hydrocortisone and other agents. *Gerontologia* 19, 138–52.

Williams, C. L., Meck, W. H., Heyer, D. D., Loy, R. 1998. Hypertrophy of basal forebrain neurons and enhanced visuospatial memory in perinatally choline-supplemented rats. *Brain Res* 794, 225–38.

Wilson, V. L., Jones, P. A. 1983. DNA methylation decreases in aging but not in immortal cells. *Science* 220, 1,055–57.

Wilson, V. L., Smith, R. A., Ma, S., Cutler, R. G. 1987. Genomic 5-methyldeoxycytidine decreases with age. *J. Biol. Chem.* 262:21, 9,948–51.

INDEX

Abbreviated methionine-loading test for plasma HCY, 20–21
Acetaldehyde, 76
Acetylcholine, 15, 48, 155, 159–60, 163–64
Adenine, 99
Adenosine triphosphate (ATP), 14
Adrenaline, 15, 155
Aging and longevity
  cataracts, 172
  choline and, 176–77
  diet and, 186
  DNA and, 180–86
  evolution and, 58–60, 177–86
  genetics and, 177–80
  graying hair, 173
  HCY, folates, and, 167–76
  homocystinuria, 170–76
  osteoporosis, 171–72
  scoliosis, 172
  skin changes, 173
AIDS, 103, 149, 150
Alcohol consumption, 76–81
Allergies, 148–49
Alpha tocopherol, 63
Alzheimer's disease, 16, 48, 164–66, 176, 177
Ames, Bruce, 129–30
Amino acids, essential, 31–32
Anemia, 13, 90–91, 146–48
  folic acid and, 51
  pregnancy and, 84–85
  vitamin B_6 and, 52
  vitamin B_{12} and, 53
  women and, 90–91

  zinc and, 54
Anencephaly, 87
Anorexia, folic acid and, 51
Anticoagulation drugs, vitamin E and, 63
Anticonvulsants, supplements and, 89
Antioxidants, 36, 55
Anxiety, supplements and, 71
Arginine, 32
Arteriosclerosis
  in children, 11–12, 108, 112–13
  HCY and, 11–12, 13, 113–19, 167–70
  methionine and, 50
Arthritis
  fish oil and, 64
  osteoarthritis, 135–36
  rheumatoid, 13, 85–86, 133–34
Asthma, 55, 148–49
Atherosclerosis, 113, 115
Attention span, vitamin B_{12} and poor, 53
Autocannibalism, 177
Autoimmune diseases, 103, 134, 136. *See also under type of*
Avocados, 30, 189–90

Bagels
  white, 39
  whole-wheat/whole-grain, 38
Barak, Anthony, 77, 78, 127
Bases, 99–100

Basil Red Pepper Salad Dressing, 224–25
Beans, 33, 190–91
Betaine
    alcohol and, 77–78
    cancer and, 127
    homocystinuria and, 109–10
    role of, 49–50
    as a supplement, 60
    well-being and, 158
Beta tocopherol, 63
Birth defects, 13, 19, 87–88
    folic acid and, 51
Blood clotting, HCY and, 117–18
Blood tests
    abbreviated methionine-loading test for plasma HCY, 20–21
    fasting plasma homocysteine test, 18–19
    HCY thiolactone test, 22
    for measuring levels of DNA methylation, 22–23
    for measuring levels of SAM, 22
Blood vessels, damage to, 11
Blueberry Pancakes, 210–11
Body mass index (BMI), 73
Breads
    not recommended, 197
    recommended, 196–97
    white, 39
    whole-wheat/whole-grain, 38
Breakfast recipes, 209–11
Breast cancer, vitamin E and, 63
Burrito, 212–13
Butterfat, 28, 31

Cabbage Salad, 223–24
CAF1 (carbohydrates as fiber) symbol, 29, 42–44
CAF2 (calories as fat) symbol, 29, 44–46
Cancer
    choline and, 125–26, 132
    DNA methylation and, 104, 124–32
    folic acid and, 128, 129–30

nutrition and, 125–26
    preventing and treating, 127–32
    selenium and, 55
    supplements and, 62–63, 70
    vitamin E and, 62–63
Canned foods
    acceptable, 192
    highly recommended, 190–91
    not recommended, 192–93
    recommended, 191–92
Canola oil, 27, 28, 29
Carbohydrates
    acceptable sources, 38–39
    not recommended sources, 39–40
    recommended sources, 35–38
    role of, 35
Carnitine, 15
Carotid artery wall thickening, 116–17
Carpal tunnel syndrome, vitamin B_6 and, 52
Cataracts, 16, 110, 172
CD4+ T-cell immunodeficiency, 103
Cell amnesia, 101
Cell membrane fluidity
    methylation, 96–98
    how it works, 96–98
Cereals, 205–06, 210
Cerebrospinal fluid, 14, 97, 140–41, 145
Cervical dysplasia
    folic acid and, 51
    supplements and, 91–92
CG islands, 185
Cheeses, 34, 203, 204
Chicken, protein in, 33
Chicken vegetable soup, 47
Chicken with Salad or Steamed Veggies, 213
Chili, 47–48, 191
Cholestasis, 16, 85
Cholesterol, 97, 113
Choline
    aging/longevity and, 176–77

Alzheimer's disease and, 165
cancer and deficiency in, 125–26, 132
during embryonic and new-born development, 89–90
exercise and, 73–74
mental functions and, 163–64
role of, 36, 48–49
as a supplement, 60–61
Chondrocytes, 135
Chromosomes, 100
Chronic fatigue syndrome (CFS), 141–43, 151
Cirrhosis of the liver, 77
Clarke, Steven, 106–07
Cobalamin, 53
   See also Vitamin B$_{12}$
Coconut oil, 28, 31
Colon cancer, 31, 125, 128–29
folic acid and, 51
Condiments, 193
Convulsions, supplements and, 72
Cookies, 39, 200–1
Corn, 39
Corn oil, 28, 30
Cottonseed oil, 28, 30
Crackers
recommended and not recommended, 198
white, 39
whole-wheat/whole-grain, 38
Cream, 31
Creatine, 15
Crohn's disease, 148
Cystadane, 110
Cysteine, 52, 54, 56, 67
Cytidine 5'-diphosphocholine (CDP-choline), 165
Cytosine, 99

Dairy products
acceptable, 204
no-fat, 34
not recommended, 204
recommended, 203–4
Deli food, 205
Delta tocopherol, 63

Dementia, vitamin B$_{12}$ and, 53
Depression
folic acid and, 51, 157–58
HCY and, 7, 13
postpartum, 86
SAM and, 16, 155–60
supplements and manic, 70–71
vitamin B$_{12}$ and, 53
in women, 92
Dermatitis, vitamin B$_6$ and, 52
Desserts, 206–7
DHA (docosahexaenoic acid), 64
Diabetes
fish oil and, 64
HCY and, 120
Diarrhea, folic acid and, 51
Dietary methyl deficiency, 143
Diet tips. *See* Food types
Dips, 195–96, 225–26
DNA methylation
aging/longevity and, 180–86
cancer and, 104, 124–32
folic acid and, 51
gender differences, 83
lupus and, 136–38
methyltransferase, 102–6
protection and maintenance of, 7–8
rheumatoid arthritis and, 133–34
role of, 99–106
SAM and, 16
tests for measuring, 22–23
zinc and, 54
Dopamine, 15, 155
Down's syndrome, 117
Drinks, recommended and not recommended, 207–8
Dry foods
acceptable, 192
highly recommended, 190–91
not recommended, 192–93
recommended, 191–92
Dwarfism, zinc and, 54

Eggs, protein in, 34
Elavil, 140

Embryonic stem (ES) cells, 105
Encephalocele, 87
Endogenous retroviruses (ERVs), 103–4
Endothelial cells, 114
EPA (eicosopentaenoic acid), 64
Epilepsy, supplements and, 72
Epstein-Barr virus, 142
Estrogen, 7, 15, 83, 94
Ethionine, 126
Exercise, 73–75
Eye disorders, 11

Fasting plasma homocysteine test, 18–19
Fats
    acceptable sources, 30
    comparison of dietary, 26–29
    mobilization of, 98
    monounsaturated, 27–29
    not recommended sources, 30–31
    polyunsaturated, 27–29
    recommended sources, 29–30
    saturated, 27–29
Fibroblasts, 181
Fibrocystic breast disease, vitamin E and, 63
Fibromyalgia, 139–41
Fish
    fat in, 27, 28–29, 30
    protein in, 32
    recipes, 213–16
    recommended, 201
Fish and Vegetable Curry, 215
Fish oil, 64
Fish with Salad or Steamed Veggies, 213
5-azacytidine, 104
Flour, white, 39
Fluoxetine, 157–58
Folates. See Folic acid
Folic acid (FA)
    aging/longevity and, 167–76
    alcohol and, 76–77
    cancer and, 128, 129–30
    depression and, 51, 157–58
    heart attack, alcohol, and, 78–80

pregnancy and, 84–85, 87–88
    role of, 36, 51–52, 67, 98–99
    as a supplement, 61–62
    testing for, 21
    toxicity of, 61–62
Food pyramid, 41
Food types
    guidelines/tips, 40–42
    proportions guideline, 42–46
Framingham Heart Study, 118–19
Frozen foods, recommended and not recommended, 204–5
Fruits
    carbohydrates in, 37–38
    recommended, 189

Gamma tocopherol, 63
Gene expression, 6, 100–1
Genetic methyl deficiency, 143
Genetics
    aging/longevity and, 177–80
    HCY and, 120–21
Glucosamine sulfate, 136
Glycine, 49
G-proteins, 16
Graded effect, 118
Graves' disease, 103
Graying hair, 173
Guanine, 99

Hayflick, Leonard, 180–81
HCY. See Homocysteine
Headache, folic acid and, 51
Healing ability, zinc and, 54
Health Professionals Follow-Up Study, 128
Heart attack, alcohol and, 78–80
Heart disease
    betaine and, 49
    in children, 112–13
    folic acid and, 51
    HCY and, 13, 14, 113–19
    lupus and, 93
    selenium and, 55
    women and, 95
Heart palpitations, folic acid and, 51

Hemorrhaging, fish oil and, 64
Heterozygotes, 105
High-pressure liquid chro-
    matography (HPLC), 18
Histamine, 7, 15, 148, 155
Histamine N-methyltransferase
    (HMT), 148
Histidine, 32
HIV, 149–51
Homocysteine (HCY)
    abbreviated methionine-
        loading test for plasma
        HCY, 20–21
    aging/longevity and, 167–76
    factors affecting levels of,
        120–21
    fasting plasma homocysteine
        test, 18–19
    heart disease/stroke and,
        113–19
    lowering, 121–23
    normal range for, 19, 20, 168
    in pregnant women, 19
    role of, 10–14
    schizophrenia and, 160–62
    supplements and, 121–23,
        158–59, 174
    testing for, 18–22
    thiolactone test, 22
Homocystinuria, 11–12, 49, 94,
    108–11, 113
    aging/longevity and, 170–76
Homozygotes, 105
Hordaland Homocysteine Study,
    73, 94, 118–19
Hormone replacement therapy
    (HRT), 94
Hostility, folic acid and, 51
Hot dogs, 34, 212
How and Why We Age (Hayflick),
    181
Human endogenous retrovirus
    (HERV), 103
Human Nutrition Research Cen-
    ter on Aging (HNRCA), 134
Human papillomavirus (HPV-
    16), 91
Human studies, 107–11
Hummus Dip, 225

Hydralazine, 137
    Hydrogenated oils, 26–30
Hyperhomocysteinemia, 12–13,
    108, 113, 120

Ice cream, 31
Inborn errors of metabolism,
    112–13
Inflammatory disorders, fish oil
    and, 64
Influenza, 151
Inositol
    neural tube defects and, 88
    role of, 56
    as a supplement, 65
Insomnia, supplements and, 71
Iron, 62, 64, 90–91, 146–47
Isoleucine, 32

Kagan, B. L., 156, 157
Kidney failure, HCY and, 120
Kim's Chili, 216–17
Knockout mice studies, 104–7

Lard, 28, 31
L-dopa, 71
Lecithin. See Phosphatidyl-
    choline
Lethargy, zinc and, 54
Leucine, 32
Life Extension Foundation, 69,
    228
Lips, vitamin B_6 and cracked, 52
Little Rock Catfish, 214
Liver disease, 16, 77–78
Longevity. See Aging and
    longevity
Lupus, 92–93, 136–38
Lymphocytes, 93
Lympholeukemia, 124
Lysine, 32

Macronutrients, 31
Maintenance methylation, 102
Manic depression, supplements
    and, 70–71
Margarines, 29, 30
Mayonnaise, 194–96
McCully, Kilmer S., 12, 112–13

Meat
  acceptable, 202
  not recommended, 203
  protein in, 32, 34
  recommended, 201–2
Megaloblastic anemia, 84–85
Melatonin, 7, 15, 96
Memory, 4
  acetylcholine and choline
    and, 163–64
  folic acid and, 51
Menopause, 93–94
Mental function, acetylcholine
  and choline and, 163–164
Mental problems
  See also Depression
  Alzheimer's disease, 16, 48,
    164–66, 176, 177
  schizophrenia, 160–63
Mental retardation, 11, 109
  betaine and, 49
  Down's syndrome, 117
Methionine, 14
  methionine-loading tests for
    plasma HCY, 20–21, 134,
    153
  cancer and deficiency in,
    125–26, 128–29
  HIV and, 151
  protein and, 31–32, 74–75
  role of, 50, 67, 99
  schizophrenia and, 160–61
  as a supplement, 65–66,
    74–75
Methotrexate, 134
Methylation
  defined, 5–9
  diseases associated with low,
    7
  human studies, 107–11
  knockout mice studies,
    104–7
  maintenance of DNA, 102
Methylation Research Institute,
  227
Methylenetetrahydrofolate
  reductase (MTHFR), 162
Methyl groups, defined, 2, 6
Methyl malonic acid (MMA), 21

Methyl metabolism, 6
Micromolar, 12
Milk
  low-fat, 34, 204
  skim, 34, 203
  whole, 34, 204
Miscarriage, 13, 19, 88
Miso Soup, 222–23
Mitrochondria, 15
Monocytes, 137
Mononucleosis, 151
Monounsaturated fat, 27–29
Mulligatawny Stew, 217–18
Multiple sclerosis (MS), 53, 86,
  143–46
Mycoplasma, 151
Myelin basic protein, 8, 16, 143,
  144
Myelin sheath, 86, 143–44,
  149

N-acetylserotonin, 155
National Cancer Institute,
  182–83
National Institutes of Aging,
  182–83
Nature's Plus, 69
Nature's Way, 69
Nervous system disorders
  chronic fatigue syndrome,
    141–43
  fibromyalgia, 139–41
  multiple sclerosis, 53, 86,
    143–46
Neural tube defects (NTDs),
  folic acid and, 51, 87–88
Neurons, 163
Neurotransmitters, 7, 96, 154
  See also under type of
Nonsteroidal anti-inflammatory
  drugs (NSAIDs), 136
Nortriptyline, 158
Nurses Health Study, 128, 129
Nutritional deficiencies
  cancer and, 125–26
  HCY and, 121
Nutrition Facts labels, under-
  standing, 42–46
Nuts, 27, 30, 192

Oakley, Godfrey, 88
Oatmeal, 39
Oceanside Tacos, 221–22
Oils
  See also under type of
  acceptable, 194
  not recommended, 194
  recommended, 193–94
Olive oil, 28, 30
Olives, 30
Omega-3 polyunsaturated fatty
  acids, 27, 64
Oncogenes, 13, 127
Oral contraceptives, 93
Orleans-Madras Hot Fish,
  213–14
Ornish, Dean, 35
Osteoarthritis, 135–36
Osteoporosis, 11, 16, 94, 171–72
  betaine and, 49

Pain reliever, SAM as, 16
Palm oil, 28, 30
Paranoia, folic acid and, 51
Parkinson's disease, supple-
  ments and, 71
Partially hydrogenated oils. *See*
  Hydrogenated oils
Pasta, 39, 197
Pasta with "Alfredo" Sauce,
  218–19
Pasta with Tomato Sauce,
  219–20
Peanut butter, 30
Peanuts, 28, 30
Peas, 190
Peripheral vascular disease, 13
p53 gene, 125
Phenylalanine, 32
Phosphatidylcholine (lecithin),
  15, 48, 144, 155, 163, 165
Phosphatidylethanolamine, 163
Phospholipids, 98
Physicians Health Study,
  118–119
Phytochemicals, 35–36
Pizza, 220–21
Polyunsaturated fat, 27–29
Popcorn, 39

Postpartum depression, 86
Potassium, 35
Potato chips, 39
Potatoes, 39
Preeclampsia, 13, 85
Pregnancy
  anemia, 84–85
  birth defects, 13, 19, 51,
    87–88
  cholestasis, 16, 85
  choline during embryonic
    and newborn development,
    89–90
  daily multivitamin program
    during, example of, 90
  folic acid and, 84–85, 87–88
  HCY and, 19
  health prior to, 88–89
  miscarriage, 13, 19, 88
  multiple sclerosis (MS), 53, 86
  postpartum depression, 86
  preeclampsia, 13, 85
  rheumatoid arthritis, 85–86
  selenium and, 55
  zinc and, 54, 55
Premenstrual syndrome (PMS)
  supplements and, 91
  vitamin E and, 63
Pritikin, Nathan, 35
Procainamide, 137
Progesterone, 94
Prostaglandins, 28, 62, 64
Protein
  acceptable sources, 34
  not recommended sources,
    34
  powders, 74
  recommended sources, 32–34
  role of, 31–32
Protein L-isoaspartyl methyltransferase (PIMT), 172
Proteoglycans, 135
Prozac, 140
Psoriasis, fish oil and, 64
Pyridoxine/pyridoxal/pyridox-
  amine, 52

Quick Spicy Fish, 215–16
Quinidine, 137

Recipes, 209–26
Refried Bean Dip and Salsa, 225
Repetitive jumping gene, 102–3
Rheumatoid arthritis, 13, 85–86, 133–34
Rice
    brown, 192
    white, 192
Richardson, Bruce, 134
Rimm, Eric, 78, 79, 95

S-adenosylhomocysteine (SAH), 13, 126
S-adenosylmethionine (SAM)
    alcohol and, 77–78
    betaine and, 77–78
    cancer and, 127
    chronic fatigue syndrome and, 142–43
    cholestasis and, 85
    depression and, 155–60
    fibromyalgia and, 140–41
    metabolism and, 67
    osteoarthritis and, 135–36
    role of, 14–17, 155
    tests for measuring, 22
Safflower oil, 28, 30
Salad dressings, 194–96, 224–25
Salads, 223–24
Salsas, 195, 225
Saturated fat, 27–29
Schizophrenia, 160–63
Scoliosis, 172
Seafood, 201
Sears, Barry, 35
Seizures, 16
    supplements and, 72
    vitamin B_6 and, 52
Selenium, 55–56, 65
Selenocysteine, 56
Selenomethionine, 56, 65
Selhub, Jacob, 116
Sertraline, 158
Sesame oil, 30
Sesame Salad Dressing, 224
Shortenings, 29, 30
Shrimp, 33, 201
Sjögren's syndrome, 103
Skin changes, aging and, 173

Smoking, 81
Smoky Toasted Fast Sandwich, 211
Snack foods, 198–200, 225–26
Soda pop, 39
Soups, 191, 192–93, 222–23
Soy-based products, protein in, 33
Soybean oil, 27, 28, 30
Soybeans, protein in, 33
Specialty Laboratories, 228
Spices, 193
Spina bifida, 87, 88
Split pea soup, 47
Stampfer, Meir, 95
Stenosis, 114–16
Sterility, zinc and, 54
Stroke
    betaine and, 49
    folic acid and, 51
    HCY and, 13, 14, 113–19
Subacute combined degeneration, 53
Sugar, refined, 39
Sunflower oil, 28, 30
Supplements
    betaine, 49–50, 60
    choline, 36, 48–49, 60–61
    diseases/conditions incompatible with taking, 70–72
    fish oil, 64
    folic acid, 21, 36, 51–52, 61–62
    inositol, 56, 65
    lowering HCY with, 122–23
    methionine, 14, 20–21, 31–32, 50, 65–66
    need to use, 58–60
    sample programs, 67–70
    selenium, 55–56, 65
    vitamin B_6, 21–22, 52–53, 62
    vitamin B_{12}, 21–22, 53–54, 62
    vitamin E, 62–64
    when and how to take, 66–67
    zinc, 54–55, 62
Swank, Roy, 145

Tacos, 221–22
T-cells, 93

Threonine, 32
Threshold effect, 118
Thrombi, 117–118
Thymine, 99
Thyroid metabolism, selenium
    and, 55
Tocopherol, 63
Trans-fatty acids, 29
Triglycerides, 78
Trimethylamine, 165
Trimethylglycine (TMG), 49–50,
    60
Tryptophan, 32
Tuna Sandwich, 46, 211–12
Turkey, protein in, 33
Twinlab, 69

Ulcerative colitis, 148

Valine, 32
Vanyushin, Boris, 182
Vascular diseases, HCY and,
    117–19
Vascular smooth muscle cells
    (VSMC), 113–14
Vegetable oils, fat in, 27
  hydrogenated/partially
    hydrogenated, 29, 30
Vegetables
  acceptable, 189–90

carbohydrates in, 35–37
not recommended, 190
recommended, 188–89
Veggie Burgers, 212
Vitamin B_6
  role of, 21–22, 52–53
  as a supplement, 62
Vitamin B_{12}
  in pregnancy, 85
  role of, 21–22, 53–54
  as a supplement, 62
Vitamin E, 62–64
Vitamin K deficiencies, 63

Weight lifting, 74–75
White Sauce, 222
Whole-wheat/whole-grain
    foods, 38–39
Wills, Lucy, 84
Wills factor, 84

Yeast selenium, 65
Yogurt, 34, 203, 204

Zinc, 54–55, 62, 67, 91, 102
Zinc fingers, 54
Zone, The (Sears), 35